Sandhya Sharma
Charu Khurana

The Evolution of the Smile: From Survival to Significance

Sandhya Sharma
Charu Khurana

The Evolution of the Smile: From Survival to Significance

LAP LAMBERT Academic Publishing

Cover image: www.ingimage.com

Publisher:
LAP LAMBERT Academic Publishing
is a trademark of
Dodo Books Indian Ocean Ltd. and OmniScriptum S.R.L publishing group

120 High Road, East Finchley, London, N2 9ED, United Kingdom
Str. Armeneasca 28/1, office 1, Chisinau MD-2012, Republic of Moldova, Europe
Managing Directors: Ieva Konstantinova, Victoria Ursu
info@omniscriptum.com

Printed at: see last page
ISBN: 978-620-8-44404-4

The Evolution of the Smile: From Survival to Significance

About the Authors

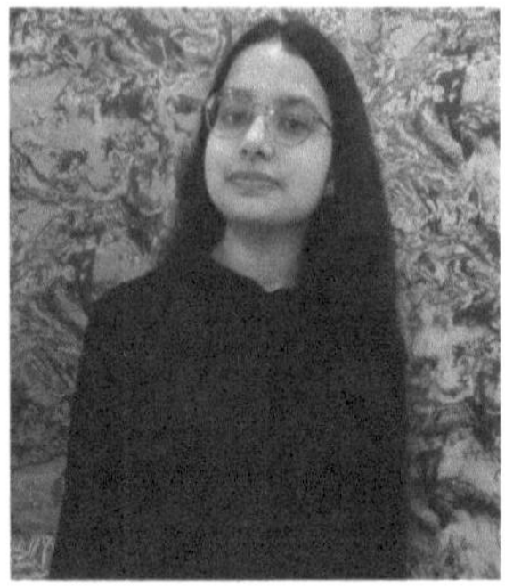

Ms. Sandhya Sharma

Sandhya Sharma is a passionate and dedicated final-year BDS student at SGT Dental College, with a keen interest in the science and evolution of the human smile. She currently serves as the secretary of an academic club. Passionate about blending research with creativity, this book reflects her curiosity and dedication to exploring the smile from both scientific and cultural perspectives.

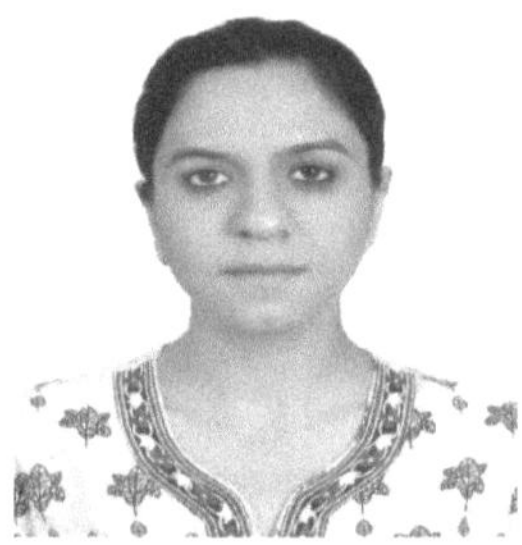

Dr. Charu Khurana

Dr. Charu Khurana is a skilled professional working as an Associate Professor and Head in the Department of public health dentistry at SGT dental College, Hospital and Research Institute, SGT University Gurugram, Haryana, India. She has an experience of more than 7 years of teaching dental undergraduate and postgraduate students in the same domain.

Content

Section: 1

Biology of teeth and Human Smile

Chapter: 1
Introduction of Human smile

For most of human history, art depicted people with solemn faces—rigid, emotionless, and carefully composed. Ancient Egyptian carvings, Mesopotamian reliefs, and early Greek statues all shared one thing in common: their subjects rarely smiled.

Then, something remarkable happened.

Around 4,500 years ago, a limestone statue of an Egyptian nobleman named *Sheikh el-Beled* broke the mold. Unlike the stiff, expressionless figures of his time, his lips curved ever so slightly, revealing what appeared to be the first recorded smile in history. But what made this smile even more fascinating was not just its presence—but what it subtly hinted at: teeth.

Fast-forward to ancient Greece, and the Archaic Smile appeared on statues of gods and mortals alike. These weren't wide, open-mouthed grins, but subtle, knowing smiles—often revealing a slight glimpse of teeth, a symbol of vitality and inner strength. In a world where most artistic expressions avoided overt emotion, the appearance of smiles with teeth suggested a shift in how humans viewed joy, confidence, and even power.

But why was smiling with teeth once so rare? And how did it evolve into the wide, bright smiles we see today? The answer lies in a fascinating journey through evolution, culture, biology, and social psychology.

From the fang-bearing grins of our primate ancestors to the dazzling Hollywood smiles of today, the way we smile—and the way we show our teeth—has transformed over millions of years. This book explores that journey, uncovering how our smiles, our teeth, and even our perceptions of beauty have shaped human history.

So, the next time you smile in the mirror, remember: your teeth tell a story—one that began long before you were born.

It is hard to picture a social interaction where none of the people involved show any emotions. Humans are inherently social creatures, and emotional expression is key to how we connect and communicate with one another. Emotions are vital for social coordination, which is essential for our survival and overall happiness.

When we engage with others, our emotions act as signals that help us convey our intentions and build connections. For example, a smile can show friendliness, while a frown may indicate discomfort. These non-verbal cues add depth to our conversations and help us understand each other better.

Additionally, sharing emotions fosters empathy and compassion. When we express our feelings, it allows others to relate to our experiences, promoting a sense of belonging and support. Without emotional expression, misunderstandings can arise, leading to feelings of isolation. Therefore, emotions are not just a part of human interaction; they are fundamental to our social lives, helping us cooperate and understand one another.

This interaction involving smiling can be understood as a form of recurrent facial mimicry, where individuals mirror each other's facial expressions. For example, when a friend greets you with a warm smile, you often find yourself smiling back without even thinking about it. This phenomenon occurs as a natural reaction to the emotional expressions observed in others, creating a cycle of mutual engagement.

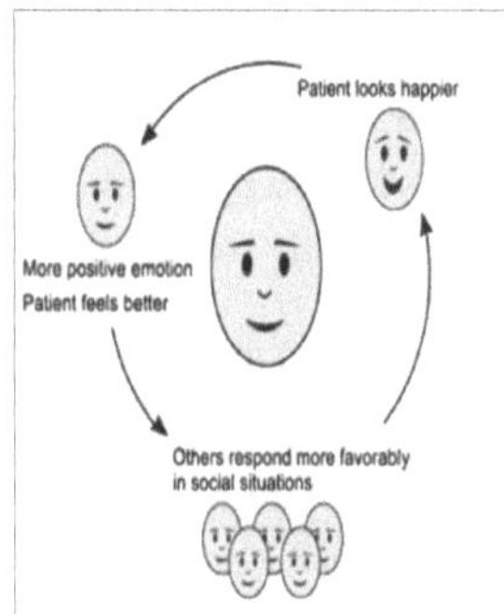

Facial mimicry plays a significant role in social interactions, as it helps to enhance emotional connection and understanding. When people unconsciously imitate each other's smiles, it fosters a sense of rapport and can lead to increased feelings of warmth and trust. Consider a scenario where a customer enters a store, and the cashier welcomes them with a genuine smile. In most cases, the customer reciprocates the smile, making the interaction more pleasant and comfortable. This mirroring effect is not limited to smiles; it can also apply to other emotional expressions, such as frowning or laughing. For instance, if a group of friends is laughing at a joke, even someone who didn't hear it might start laughing simply because of the contagious nature of the expression.

Moreover, this mimicry is not just about replicating facial expressions; it also influences our emotional states. Research has shown that when we mimic positive expressions like smiling, we can actually elevate our mood and promote a more positive atmosphere in social settings. Imagine walking into a room where everyone is cheerful and smiling—it naturally lifts your spirits and makes you feel more welcome. In essence, recurrent facial mimicry of smiling is a powerful tool for building social bonds and facilitating communication, highlighting the interconnectedness of our emotional experiences.

Everyone around you might be affected by your grin, changing their emotional and mental states. A positive feedback loop is created when you smile since it frequently inspires people to smile back. In addition to improving the environment, this engagement helps people feel more connected and like they belong, which fortifies social ties.

From a biological standpoint, smiling causes the brain to release a number of hormones, including serotonin, oxytocin, and endorphins. Endorphins are the body's natural mood enhancers and pain relievers; they lower tension and increase happiness. Often called the "love hormone," oxytocin promotes emotions of bonding and trust that can strengthen bonds and improve social ties. Another significant neurotransmitter, serotonin, is essential for controlling mood and emotional health.

Smiling causes the production of these hormones, which not only lift your spirits but also benefit people around you. Others may have comparable hormone increases in response to your grin, fostering a feeling of happiness and optimism that is shared by all. This knock-on effect can improve group dynamics and increase the satisfaction and enjoyment of social interactions. In the end, a simple grin can have a big impact, changing the emotional atmosphere of any space and strengthening social ties.

This contagious smile is backed by science. Studies reveal that seeing a smile automatically prompts our facial muscles to respond with a smile.

Now we will understand the different muscles involved in producing this universal expression that transcends culture and serves as a powerful nonverbal cue to communicate.

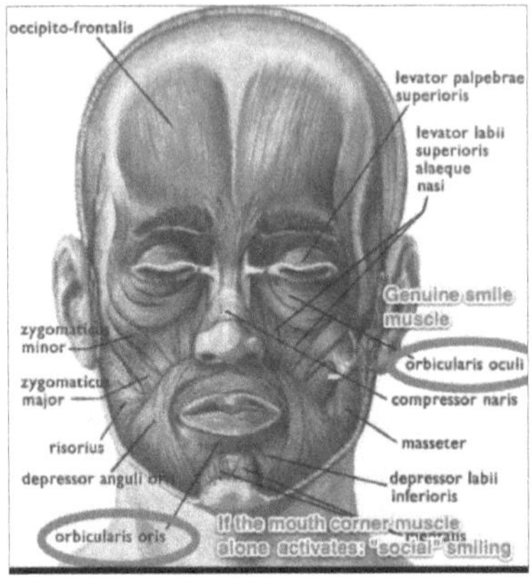

A smile is a complex facial expression produced by the coordinated movement of the perioral muscles. Gaining a deeper understanding of these muscles' roles is essential for reconstructive and aesthetic dental procedures. Rubin classified smiles into three primary types based on the dominant muscle activity: the Mona Lisa smile, the canine smile, and the full dental smile.

However, this classification relies on subjective evaluation of a person's maximum smile, lacking objective scientific validation. Moreover, the boundaries between these smile types are often indistinct, as they frequently overlap. This overlap reduces the classification's reliability and practical significance in clinical settings.

To address these limitations, advanced imaging technologies now allow for a more precise and dynamic assessment of smiling. Three-dimensional (3D) digital stereophotogrammetry has proven to be an effective tool for analyzing smile mechanics in real-time. Research using this technology has examined various aspects, including the extent and speed of muscle movement, smile symmetry, changes in the surface area of the oral region, and movement vector analysis. These objective evaluations offer a more accurate and detailed understanding of smile dynamics, enhancing both clinical applications and scientific research.

The zygomaticus major muscle serves as the primary initiator of most smiles, playing a dominant role in the initial phase of smile formation. However, the dynamics of smiling involve the coordinated activity of multiple perioral muscles beyond the zygomaticus major. Other key muscles contributing to smile expression include the levator anguli oris, which elevates the corners of the mouth; the buccinator and risorius, which assist in lateral expansion of the smile; and the depressor anguli oris, which influences the downward movement of the mouth corners. Additionally, the upward muscle group of the upper lip, including muscles such as the levator labii superioris, also plays a crucial role in modulating the smile's appearance.

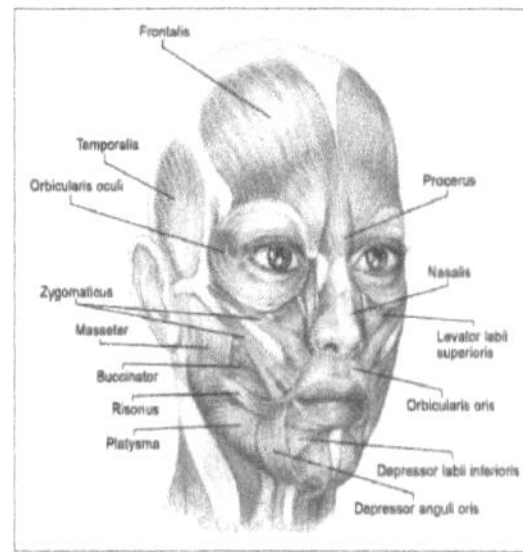

Notably, a significant proportion of smiles exhibit a mixed activation pattern, indicating that smiling is not solely dependent on a single muscle but rather on the synergistic interplay of multiple muscle groups. This suggests that the mechanism of smiling is highly individualized and complex, involving varying degrees of muscle coordination to achieve different smile expressions. Understanding these variations is essential for clinical applications, including facial reconstruction, aesthetic dentistry, and neuromuscular rehabilitation.

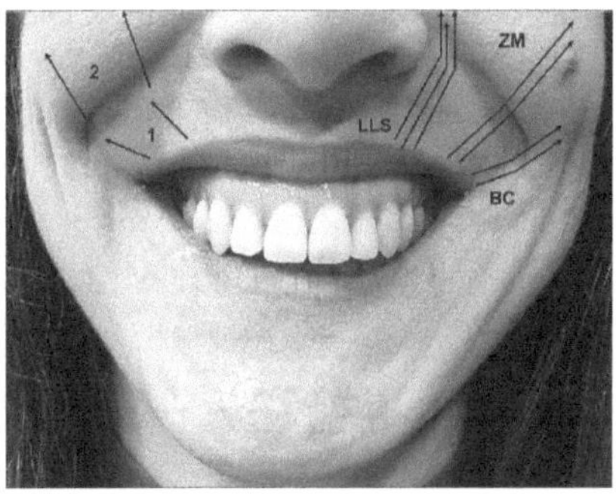

Different muscles involved during a maximum smile. The superior lip and the fold raise due to the action of three different muscle groups: The levator labii superioris (LLS), zygomaticus major (ZM), and superior fibers of the buccinator (BC)

The intricate relationship between facial muscles and emotional regulation highlights the significance of the facial feedback hypothesis, wherein the activation of specific muscles involved in smiling influences neural pathways linked to mood and stress regulation. The primary muscles responsible for smiling, such as the zygomaticus major and minor, along with associated perioral muscles, contract in response to facial nerve stimulation, lifting the corners of the mouth and altering facial expression. This muscular activity is not merely a mechanical process; it also initiates afferent feedback to the brain, particularly targeting regions like the limbic system and hypothalamus, which govern emotional responses. By stimulating these neural circuits, smiling—whether voluntary or spontaneous—triggers the release of endorphins, which serve as natural mood enhancers and stress regulators. Consequently, the neuromuscular activation of a smile extends beyond aesthetics, playing a critical role in both psychological well-being and physiological homeostasis, demonstrating the profound interconnectedness of facial musculature, neurochemistry, and emotional health.

Facial expressions, particularly smiling, can influence emotional states by engaging neural pathways associated with mood regulation. Research led by Sarah Pressman, Ph.D., at the University of Kansas highlights the bidirectional relationship between facial muscle activation and emotional perception. While it is well established that positive emotions naturally induce smiling, the inverse is also true—intentionally activating the muscles involved in smiling can generate a sensation of happiness. This phenomenon is attributed to the brain interpreting the physical act of smiling as a genuine emotional response, thereby triggering neurochemical changes.

Smiling engages the facial nerve (cranial nerve VII), which innervates various muscles responsible for facial expressions. When these muscles contract, they send afferent feedback to the brain, particularly to the limbic system, which is responsible for emotion regulation. This neural signaling stimulates the release of endorphins, which are opioid-like neuropeptides secreted by the pituitary gland and the hypothalamus. Endorphins bind to opiate receptors in the brain and spinal cord, acting as natural analgesics and mood enhancers. These neurochemicals play a crucial role in reducing pain perception, alleviating stress, and promoting a sense of well-being.

Furthermore, the release of endorphins has physiological effects beyond mood enhancement. By reducing the body's stress response, smiling indirectly influences the autonomic nervous system, particularly the parasympathetic nervous system, which helps regulate heart rate and blood pressure. When an individual experiences positive emotion—either genuinely or as a result of facial feedback—the body experiences reduced cortisol levels and an increase in vagal tone, which promotes relaxation and cardiovascular stability.

This mechanism explains why seemingly trivial actions, such as smiling at an image of a puppy or a comforting memory, can induce a sense of happiness and reduce physiological stress. The facial feedback hypothesis suggests that these neurophysiological responses reinforce the link between facial expressions and emotional experiences, offering potential applications in psychological and stress management interventions.

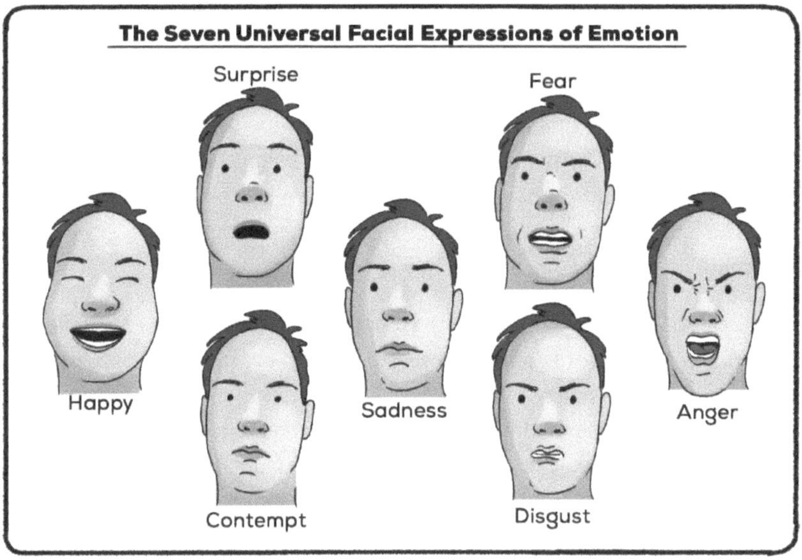

The brain is inherently programmed to control facial muscles in distinct patterns to convey emotions. When these muscles contract, they exert tension on the skin, enabling the formation of a wide range of expressions, including frowning, smiling, raising an eyebrow, and winking. Remarkably, humans can generate thousands of unique facial expressions, each varying in duration from as brief as 0.5 seconds (microexpressions) to up to 4 seconds.

Types of Smiles

The brain's ability to regulate facial muscles for emotional expression is fundamental in shaping the different types of smiles observed in human interactions. Facial expressions result from the coordinated contraction of various perioral muscles, allowing for a diverse range of smiles that reflect subtle emotional nuances. Given that humans are capable of producing thousands of facial expressions, the degree of muscle activation and involvement determines the specific type of smile displayed.

One of the most well-known classifications of smiles was proposed by Rubin, who categorized them into three distinct types based on the dominant muscle movements:

1. Mona Lisa Smile – This type of smile is characterized by a subtle and restrained expression, primarily involving minimal engagement of the zygomaticus major. The corners of the mouth are gently elevated, while the upper lip remains largely inactive, creating a mysterious or reserved appearance. The orbicularis oculi

may be slightly involved, producing faint crow's feet at the outer corners of the eyes, often associated with a genuine yet controlled smile.

2. Canine Smile – In this type, the levator labii superioris and levator anguli oris muscles contract, lifting the upper lip and exposing the canine teeth. This smile conveys confidence or playfulness and is commonly observed in both social and expressive contexts. The prominence of the canines gives this smile a distinct, sometimes mischievous or assertive appearance.

3. Full Dental Smile – This is the most expressive form, where multiple muscles, including the zygomaticus major, orbicularis oculi, levator anguli oris, and others, work in synergy to produce a broad smile. The lips retract widely, exposing both upper and lower teeth. The engagement of the orbicularis oculi in a genuine full smile creates noticeable eye crinkles, also known as Duchenne markers, which are associated with authentic happiness and joy.

Research literature suggests that humans are capable of producing approximately 19 distinct types of smiles, yet only a subset—around five—are associated with genuine happiness and subjective well-being (Gorvett, 2017). Each type of smile serves a unique communicative function, reinforcing emotional expression and interpersonal connections. Smiling is not only an indicator of emotional states but also plays a role in social signaling, where subtle variations in muscle activation convey different psychological meanings.

According to Ekman (1993), the following types of smiles are commonly associated with positive emotions and overall well-being:

1. Duchenne Smile – The Smile of True Happiness

The Duchenne smile is widely regarded as the most authentic expression of genuine joy and positive emotion. This smile is characterized by the simultaneous activation of two key muscle groups:

- Zygomaticus major – Lifts the corners of the mouth.
- Orbicularis oculi – Engages the muscles around the eyes, leading to the formation of wrinkles known as "crow's feet" at the outer corners.

This type of smile is involuntary and spontaneous, emerging in situations where an individual experiences authentic happiness, gratitude, or deep emotional satisfaction. It is typically observed in genuine social interactions, such as sharing a joyful moment with loved ones, and has been linked to positive psychological well-being, reduced stress, and enhanced social bonding.

2. Fake Smile – A Masked Expression of Happiness

A fake smile, also known as a non-Duchenne smile, is a deliberate or forced expression that does not reflect true emotional happiness. Unlike the Duchenne smile, a fake smile only involves the zygomaticus major, lifting the corners of the mouth, but lacks engagement of the orbicularis oculi, leaving the eyes unchanged.

Since the eyes are critical in expressing genuine emotions, a fake smile often appears stiff or unnatural, failing to convey true joy. It is frequently used in socially obligatory situations, such as posing for photographs, maintaining politeness in professional settings, or masking negative emotions in social interactions.

3. Uncomfortable Smile – A Smile Concealing Discomfort

An uncomfortable smile is a facial expression that emerges when an individual attempts to hide feelings of unease or social anxiety. This type of smile often lacks full symmetry, as the individual forces the zygomaticus major to contract while experiencing internal discomfort.

It is commonly observed in:

- Situations involving awkward social encounters.
- Responses to inappropriate or intrusive questions.
- Moments where an individual wants to appear agreeable despite feeling uneasy.

Psychologically, this smile serves as a coping mechanism to diffuse social tension or mask negative emotions, allowing individuals to navigate difficult interactions while maintaining social decorum.

4. Seductive Smile – A Smile as a Social Strategy

The seductive smile is a controlled facial expression that conveys attraction and flirtation. Studies by Gorvett (2017) suggest that this smile is often accompanied by:

- Sustained eye contact, which creates a sense of intimacy.
- A slow glance away, adding an element of mystery or intrigue.
- Subtle lip movements or a slight head tilt, which can enhance the expression's effectiveness.

This smile can be either dominant or submissive, depending on the context. A dominant seductive smile may be used to project confidence, while a submissive version may signal receptiveness or playfulness. The seductive smile functions as a nonverbal cue in social and romantic interactions, influencing interpersonal dynamics and attraction.

5. Sarcastic Smile – A Blend of Amusement and Contempt

A sarcastic smile is a complex expression that conveys both amusement and underlying negativity, often in the form of irony or passive aggression. This smile is typically characterized by:

- An upward movement of the mouth, similar to a genuine smile.
- A contrasting expression in the eyes, which may appear disengaged, unimpressed, or condescending.

The disparity between the lower and upper facial expressions is what distinguishes sarcasm from true amusement. This smile is often observed in situations where individuals use mock appreciation, satire, or veiled criticism, making it a common expression in humorous, competitive, or tense social exchanges.

The intersection of biology, culture, and psychology

The human smile is more than just an expression; it is a product of biological evolution, cultural shaping, and psychological significance. The way we smile and perceive smiles has been influenced by evolutionary adaptations, societal expectations, and psychological mechanisms that govern social interactions.

Biological Basis of Smiling and Teeth

From an evolutionary standpoint, smiling is deeply rooted in human survival and social bonding. Non-human primates, such as chimpanzees, display fear grins or submissive smiles to avoid conflict and establish group hierarchy. Early human ancestors, like Australopithecus, had large jaws and teeth adapted for a plant-based diet, but as Homo sapiens evolved, changes in diet led to smaller jaws and more uniform teeth . Smiling, in turn, became a crucial social tool for non-verbal communication, allowing early humans to signal friendliness and trustworthiness. The facial feedback hypothesis suggests that smiling can trigger the release of dopamine and serotonin, reinforcing positive emotions.

Cultural Variations in Smiling and Dental Aesthetics

Cultural perceptions of smiling vary significantly across societies. In Western cultures, a broad, toothy smile is associated with warmth, confidence, and openness. Conversely, in East Asian cultures, people tend to suppress overt smiling in formal settings, as it may be perceived as a sign of nervousness or insincerity. The importance of dental aesthetics also differs across societies. In Japan, "yaeba" (slightly crooked teeth) is sometimes considered attractive, whereas in the United States, straight, white teeth are seen as a marker of social status and good health.

Modern dental advancements have reinforced cultural ideals of beauty. The rise of orthodontics and cosmetic dentistry reflects how humans have moved beyond biological necessity to shape their smiles according to cultural standards. The "Hollywood smile", characterized by perfectly aligned and whitened teeth, has become a global phenomenon, influencing dental practices worldwide.

Psychological Implications of Smiling and Dental Appearance

Smiling not only reflects emotions but also influences psychological well-being. Studies show that smiling enhances mood, reduces stress, and increases social likability. In contrast, individuals with dental imperfections often experience lower self-esteem and social anxiety, particularly in cultures that emphasize perfect teeth.

Moreover, smiling plays a crucial role in first impressions. People with healthy, symmetrical teeth are perceived as more attractive, successful, and trustworthy. The halo effect—where one positive attribute (such as a beautiful smile) influences overall perception—demonstrates how deeply ingrained our biases are in human psychology.

Even in business and leadership, smiling has a significant impact. Leaders who smile are viewed as more competent and approachable, while those who rarely smile may be seen as cold or untrustworthy (14). The use of smiling in marketing, particularly in advertisements, also reinforces positive emotional associations with brands and products

The intersection of biology, culture, and psychology shapes how we perceive and use smiles. While biological evolution provided humans with the ability to smile, cultural expectations have dictated how and when we do it, and psychological mechanisms reinforce its emotional and social benefits. Understanding this complex interplay not only enhances our appreciation of human expression but also highlights how something as simple as a smile carries deep-rooted biological and social significance.

Chapter: 2

Development And Evolution of human teeth

Millions of years ago, deep in the forests of Africa, an early primate plucked a fruit from a tree and bit into it. The sound of crunching echoed through the air—a simple act of survival, but one that carried the weight of evolution. That bite, and countless others like it, would shape the human species in ways few could have imagined.

Our teeth are like time capsules, preserving the story of our ancestors. They tell us what our predecessors ate, how they lived, and even how they died. Fossilized jaws reveal a remarkable transformation: from the razor-sharp canines of early primates to the balanced, versatile teeth of modern humans. Each shift in tooth shape and function reflects an evolutionary leap—a change driven by environment, diet, and survival needs.

But how did we go from the massive, grinding molars of herbivorous apes to the smaller, well-aligned teeth of today? And what do these changes say about the way we evolved, not just biologically, but socially and culturally?

To answer these questions, we must journey back millions of years to explore how human teeth have adapted—from the thick enamel of our earliest ancestors to the straight, uniform smiles we now strive for in the modern age.

Evolution and the Role of Human Dentition

Evolution refers to the slow and continuous transformation of inherited traits within human populations over successive generations. This process is fundamental to the development of biological diversity across all forms of life. In the mid-19th century, Charles Darwin introduced the concept of natural selection, proposing that evolution occurs because organisms produce more offspring than can survive in a given environment. Those with favorable traits have a higher chance of survival and reproduction, passing these advantageous characteristics to future generations.

Scientific research suggests that all living organisms on Earth share a common ancestor, known as the Last Universal Common Ancestor (LUCA). Evolution is a fundamental principle of modern science, reinforced by extensive evidence across multiple disciplines, including biology, anthropology, psychology, astrophysics, chemistry, geology, physics, and mathematics. Additionally, behavioral and social sciences contribute to a deeper understanding of human evolutionary patterns and adaptations.

From an anthropological perspective, the study of teeth provides critical insights into human evolution. Dental structures offer valuable evidence of ancestral diets, genetic heritage, and environmental adaptations over time. Because teeth are among the most durable structures in the human body, they remain well-preserved in fossil records, making them essential for evolutionary and comparative population studies.

Certain dental traits exhibit genetic and population-specific variations, enabling scientists to trace ancestry and migration patterns. Some of the most significant dental characteristics include:

- Shovel-shaped incisors – commonly found among East Asian and Native American populations.
- Carabelli's cusp – a genetic dental feature frequently seen in European populations.
- Hypocone – an additional molar cusp significant in tracing evolutionary changes.
- Peg-shaped teeth – a variation often linked to specific ethnic groups.

These distinctive dental markers help researchers classify different populations and understand how genetic traits have evolved over centuries.

The Role of Dentition in Identification

In forensic science, dentition plays a vital role in personal identification. Every individual has a unique dental structure, ensuring that no two people, not even identical twins, have the same set of teeth. This uniqueness makes dental analysis a powerful tool for forensic identification. Various dental features contribute to individual recognition, including:

- Tooth shape and morphology – variations in size, structure, and arrangement.
- Enamel color and texture – providing clues about age, diet, and health.
- Wear patterns – revealing lifestyle habits and dietary influences.
- Dental anomalies – irregularities that aid in distinguishing individuals.

Teeth are composed of the hardest substance in the human body, allowing them to endure extreme conditions, including high temperatures, chemical exposure, and physical trauma. Because of their resilience, dental remains are often crucial in forensic investigations where other biological materials have deteriorated.

Forensic odontologists work closely with dental anthropologists and forensic experts to analyze various dental characteristics, assisting in age estimation, sex determination, ethnic origin identification, bite mark analysis, and dental record comparisons. These techniques are widely applied in criminal investigations, disaster victim identification, and missing person cases.

Development of tooth

The earliest vertebrates lacked jaws; known as agnathans. The jawed vertebrates represent pivotal advancement and proven to be more evolutionarily successful. The significant milestone in the evolution of head was the development of specialised dentition. Odontodes (teeth or toothlike structures) that have been lost in certain evolutionary lineages are pervasive among vertebrates. Most fishes, reptiles and many amphibians have polyodont, homodont and polyphyodont dentition and are composed of enamel and dentin. These teeth lack roots and are directly anchored to the bone via ankylosis and fibrous connective tissue. Mammalian dentition has roots which is ligated to alveolar bone via periodontal fibres. The detailed evolution of teeth in vertebrates is discussed later in this chapter.

Before moving ahead, it is crucial to explore the stages and molecular basis of tooth development.

Stages of tooth development

The formation of teeth is a multifaceted process that involves interaction between ectoderm of the oral cavity which generate cells responsible for enamel production and neural crest cells, which generate other structures of the tooth. The tooth germ starts growing during the first six weeks of intrauterine life, followed by laid down enamel and dentin matrix.

Various signaling pathways like Wnt, BMP, FGF, Shh and EDA plays an inevitable role in tooth development via: Initiation, Budding, Morphogenesis

There are four stages in the development of tooth germ. These include

1. Bud stage.
2. Cap stage
3. Early bell stage
4. Late bell stage

Primary epithelial band which is formed around sixth week of intrauterine life is a thickened continuous band of oral epithelium that invades underlying ectomesenchyme. This band later (seventh week) divides into dental lamina and vestibular lamina. Dental lamina contributes in the process of teeth development whereas vestibular lamina is responsible for formation of oral vestibule.

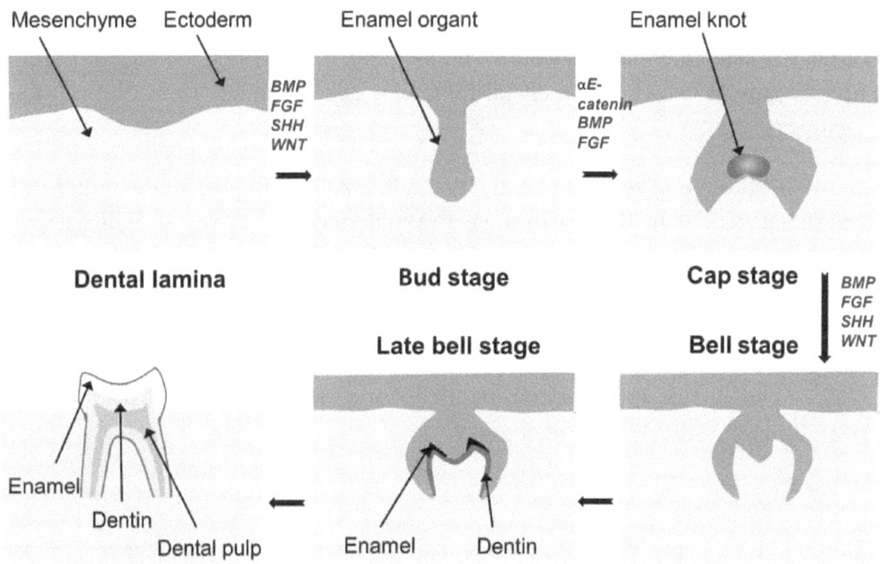

A schematic presentation of developmental stages of tooth germ.

1. Bud stage

This stage begins in the eighth week of intrauterine life characterised by swellings of enamel organ formed by dental lamina. These swellings arise at 10 distinct points indicating the future position of deciduous teeth. This stage is influenced by factors like BMP, FGF, SHH.

2. Cap stage

This stage is characterized by the growth and expansion of the enamel organ, leading to the formation of a concavity on its inner surface. As development progresses, around the 12th week of intrauterine life—during the late cap stage—the inner enamel epithelium emerges from the cuboidal cells within the enamel organ. Unlike the cuboidal cells of the enamel organ, the inner enamel epithelium cells adopt a columnar shape. This layer determines the crown's shape and later differentiates into ameloblasts, which are responsible for enamel formation. Meanwhile, the outer layer of the enamel organ develops into the outer enamel epithelium, retaining its cuboidal shape and maintaining the structure of the enamel organ.

Beneath the inner enamel epithelium, condensed mesenchymal cells give rise to the dental papilla, which later develops into the pulp. Surrounding the enamel organ is a fibrous capsule known as the dental follicle, which eventually forms the periodontal ligament.

By the 14th week of intrauterine life, two additional layers, the stratum intermedium and stellate reticulum, become distinct. The stratum intermedium, positioned above the inner enamel epithelium, consists of two to three layers of cells that facilitate the transport of nutrients to and from the ameloblasts, the enamel-forming cells. The stellate reticulum, located between the stratum intermedium and the outer enamel epithelium, is composed of star-shaped cells, from which it derives its name. This layer plays a crucial role in protecting the underlying dental tissues and maintaining the overall shape of the developing tooth

3. Bell stage

During the bell stage of tooth development, the dental lamina disintegrates, preparing for the formation of hard dental tissues. This stage marks the transition to dentinogenesis and amelogenesis, leading to the formation of dentin and enamel.

Dentin Formation (Dentinogenesis)

Cells from the inner enamel epithelium induce peripheral dental papilla cells to differentiate into odontoblasts, which secrete an unmineralized dentin matrix called predentin. Once predentin reaches approximately 5 μm in thickness, mineralization begins at random points, forming calcospherites—spherical zones of hydroxyapatite. As these fuse, they create mineralized dentin. The first-formed mineralized dentin is known as mantle dentin, while the rest is termed circumpulpal dentin. As odontoblasts deposit dentin, they retreat toward the dental papilla, leaving behind odontoblast processes, which become enclosed within dentinal tubules.

Enamel Formation (Amelogenesis)

Enamel formation begins immediately after dentin deposition. Ameloblasts, derived from the inner enamel epithelium, secrete the enamel matrix through Tomes' process at the amelodentinal junction. Mineralization starts as calcium and phosphate ions crystallize into hydroxyapatite. As more enamel matrix is secreted and mineralized, ameloblasts move outward, forming enamel prisms (rods) that extend from the amelodentinal junction to the enamel surface. As enamel matures, its mineral content increases while organic content decreases. Once enamel formation is complete, ameloblasts lose Tomes' process and become reduced enamel epithelium, which later forms the junctional epithelium after eruption.

Root Formation

After crown development, Hertwig's epithelial root sheath (HERS)—derived from the inner and outer enamel epithelium—extends apically, enclosing the dental papilla and shaping the root. The surrounding dental follicle later differentiates into the periodontal ligament (PDL) and cementum.

Cementum Formation (Cementogenesis)

Following root development, HERS undergoes fragmentation, allowing dental follicle cells to contact the root dentin. These cells differentiate into cementoblasts, which secrete cementum matrix. Mineralization follows, depositing hydroxyapatite crystals. The initial unmineralized cementum layer is called cementoid.

Periodontal Ligament (PDL) Formation

Fibroblasts within the dental follicle secrete collagen fibers, which organize into principal fibers of the PDL. As cementum forms, these fibers embed into both the cementum and the alveolar bone, creating Sharpey's fibers, which anchor the tooth within the socket and provide periodontal support.

This sequence of events ensures the proper development of teeth and their supporting structures, enabling functional occlusion and stability within the oral cavity.

Genetic and signaling

Let's make this journey more interesting by understanding the genetics and signalling in development of tooth with this epic fantasy of Kingdom of Odontia.

Once upon a time, in the vast and intricate world of Odontia, King PAX9, the great ruler of genes, sat in his crystalline throne inside the Palace of the Nucleus. Around him were his most trusted advisors—MSX1, BMP4, and FGF8, the wise architects of tooth development.

"The time has come!" King PAX9 declared. *"The first bricks of the teeth must be laid. Summon the Royal Messengers!"*

With a wave of his hand, the Signaling Messengers—WNT, BMP, SHH (Sonic Hedgehog), and FGF—rushed into the royal hall. These messengers were the most powerful communicators in Odontia, ensuring that every worker knew their task in the grand construction of teeth.

The first destination of the messengers was the land of the Oral Epithelium, where the foundation of teeth had to be laid.

- BMP and FGF messengers arrived first, carrying scrolls of instructions.
- They read aloud, *"By order of King PAX9, let the first blueprints be drawn!"*
- The epithelial builders quickly formed the dental lamina, the sacred path from which all teeth would grow.

Meanwhile, deep beneath the epithelial land, another kingdom stirred—the Ectomesenchyme, a realm of specialized workers who had migrated from the neural crest. These skilled workers were essential for shaping the tooth's internal structure.

- WNT and SHH messengers entered the ectomesenchyme kingdom and sounded the horn.
- *"Rise, mesenchymal warriors! It is time to form the tooth bud!"*
- The ectomesenchymal builders rushed forward, creating a small bud that would soon grow into a mighty tooth.

With the bud formed, the cap stage began. The messengers now had to ensure proper layering.

- BMP4 issued a decree: *"Let the enamel organ take shape!"*
- FGF called upon the mesenchymal cells: *"Form the dental papilla, the future pulp and dentin!"*
- A magical structure, the enamel knot, appeared—a tiny but powerful command center directing tooth shape!

The kingdom of Odontia marveled at the growing structure, but the greatest test was yet to come.

Now, the developing tooth resembled a bell. The final forces needed to be assembled:

- Ameloblasts were appointed as the Master Enamel Craftsmen.
- Odontoblasts became the Mighty Builders of Dentin.

Under the watchful eye of SHH and BMP, the ameloblasts laid down enamel, while the odontoblasts secreted dentin, forming the tooth's core.

As the construction neared completion, a shadow loomed over Odontia. Mutation, the Deceiver, sought to disrupt the process.

- A missing MSX1: The mesenchymal workers became confused, leading to incomplete teeth.
- A defect in PAX9: The construction of molars stopped altogether.
- Too much WNT: Extra teeth started forming, creating chaos in Odontia.

A great battle ensued. The messengers and genes worked tirelessly to correct errors, ensuring that the tooth developed smoothly. With teamwork, they defeated Mutation and restored order.

After months of labor, the first tooth was ready. The Periodontal Knights cleared the path, and with one final push, the tooth erupted into the world.

The citizens of Odontia rejoiced! The Grand Construction was a success. King PAX9 and his advisors watched with pride as the newborn tooth shone brightly, a symbol of their tireless work.

From that day on, the kingdom of Odontia continued to build, ensuring that every being had the gift of a perfect smile.

To understand the origins of teeth, it is essential to bridge the gap between their intricate development in vertebrates and their evolutionary emergence in invertebrates. The genetic signaling pathways that guide tooth development, such as BMP, FGF, and Wnt, are not exclusive to vertebrates but have deep evolutionary roots in simpler organisms. Invertebrates, particularly those with mineralized structures like mollusks and early jawless fish ancestors, exhibit primitive forms of tooth-like structures. These structures provide insight into how genetic mechanisms, initially responsible for cuticular modifications or skeletal elements, may have been co-opted and refined over time to give rise to true teeth in vertebrates. Understanding this evolutionary continuum helps trace the transition from simple biomineralized tissues to the complex dentition seen in modern species

Origin of tooth in vertebrates

Teeth are one of the most ancient and significant evolutionary adaptations in vertebrates, yet their origin remains a topic of intense scientific debate. The earliest known tooth-like structures are believed to have emerged over 500 million years ago in the posterior pharyngeal region of jawless fishes. With the rise of jawed vertebrates, teeth began to form on oral jaws, greatly enhancing their ability to capture and process food, which contributed to the widespread success of gnathostomes in both aquatic and terrestrial environments.

It remains uncertain whether teeth initially evolved alongside jaws to aid in predation and mastication or if they first developed as external dermal armor for defense against predators. Two primary hypotheses have been proposed regarding the origin of oral teeth. The "outside-in" theory suggests that teeth evolved from ectoderm-derived skin denticles that gradually folded inward and became integrated into the mouth. In contrast, the "inside-out" theory argues that teeth originated from endodermal tissues, first appearing as pharyngeal teeth in jawless vertebrates before migrating forward into the oral cavity with the evolution of jaws. However, recent research suggests that neither of these models fully explains tooth evolution.

Studies employing fate-mapping techniques in transgenic axolotls have shown that teeth can develop normally regardless of whether the oral epithelium arises from ectodermal or endodermal tissues. Additionally, experiments conducted on chicken embryos, which naturally lack the ability to form teeth, have demonstrated that mesenchyme plays a dominant role in initiating tooth development. Specifically, when neural crest cells from mice were transplanted into developing chicken embryos, they facilitated the formation of tooth germ-like structures.

Certain modern fish species, such as specific cichlids, possess both oral and pharyngeal teeth. These pharyngeal teeth develop on specialized pharyngeal jaws in regions derived from hox-positive endoderm, whereas oral teeth form in hox-negative ectodermal regions. The pharyngeal teeth found in jawless vertebrates seem to rely on an ancient genetic framework that predates the emergence of oral jaws, oral dentition, and ectodermal appendages.

During mouse development, the expression of genes like *claudin6, Foxa2, alpha-fetoprotein, Esrp1* (formerly *Rbm35a*), and *Sox2* is observed in the areas destined to become molars but not in those forming incisors. Additionally, in *Chuk*(previously known as *Ikka*) null mice, abnormal epithelial evagination occurs in incisors while molar development remains unaffected. These findings suggest variations in the epithelial origins of incisor and molar teeth, indicating distinct molecular mechanisms underlying heterodont dentition. However, despite developmental differences, both oral and pharyngeal teeth share striking similarities in their gene regulatory networks.

Research involving axolotls, cichlids, chickens, and mice collectively suggests that teeth can form despite variations in epithelial origin. These studies emphasize the critical role of mesenchyme in initiating tooth development, challenging the traditional belief that oral ectoderm is solely responsible for this process. Moreover, they highlight the conservation of gene regulatory networks across species, regardless of their germ layer origins, reinforcing the concept of deep homology in tooth evolution. Ultimately, teeth appear to have evolved through a combination of both "inside" and "outside" mechanisms, arising wherever and whenever the odontogenic-specific gene network of the mesenchyme was active.

As vertebrates conquered new ecological niches, the evolution of teeth continued to unfold in response to shifting environmental pressures. From the armored jaws of ancient placoderms to the highly specialized dentition of mammals, teeth became not only instruments of survival but also a biological archive, preserving the story of life's adaptation across millions of years.

Despite the ongoing debate between the "outside-in" and "inside-out" models of tooth evolution, one thing remains clear—teeth did not emerge as a singular, sudden innovation but rather as a gradual, complex interplay between genetic potential, developmental plasticity, and environmental demands.

The rise of early jawed vertebrates marked the beginning of a new era in dental complexity. Initially, teeth were simple, conical structures, continuously replaced throughout life. This model, seen in modern sharks, proved highly effective for grasping and tearing but lacked the efficiency of later dentitions.

As terrestrial vertebrates emerged, tooth morphology underwent a dramatic transformation. Reptilian lineages diversified, producing formidable carnivores like theropod dinosaurs with serrated, dagger-like teeth, and herbivores such as hadrosaurs with battery-like dental structures suited for grinding fibrous plant material. The ability of teeth to adapt to dietary changes became a defining characteristic of vertebrate evolution.

Mammals introduced an entirely new paradigm—**heterodonty**, the differentiation of teeth into incisors, canines, premolars, and molars. This arrangement allowed for precise processing of food, increasing digestive efficiency and supporting the metabolic demands of warm-blooded organisms. The shift from polyphyodonty (continuous tooth replacement) to diphyodonty (two sets of teeth in a lifetime) further refined occlusion, optimizing bite force and reducing tooth wear over time.

While the external morphology of teeth evolved in diverse directions, the genetic framework governing their formation remained deeply conserved across species. The same fundamental gene regulatory networks that shaped the dentition of ancient fish continue to operate in modern vertebrates.

Studies on axolotls, cichlids, and mice have demonstrated that tooth development is not solely dictated by epithelial origin but is instead orchestrated by mesenchymal signals. This suggests that teeth can form in any location where odontogenic gene expression is activated—a concept that supports the idea of deep homology in tooth evolution.

Comparative research in fish has further revealed that pharyngeal teeth, which develop from endodermal tissues, and oral teeth, derived from ectoderm, share a common genetic toolkit. This challenges the traditional dichotomy between the "inside-out" and "outside-in" models, suggesting instead that teeth arose through a combination of mechanisms, shaped by the evolutionary pressures of feeding and survival.

The evolutionary journey of teeth is far from over. As vertebrates continue to adapt to new environments and diets, dental structures will likely undergo further modifications. In humans, the rapid shift toward processed, softer foods has already influenced jaw development, leading to a higher prevalence of dental crowding and impacted wisdom teeth.

Yet, beyond natural evolution, scientific advancements in genetics and regenerative medicine may soon redefine the future of human dentition. Researchers are exploring ways to reactivate dormant tooth-regeneration pathways, potentially enabling humans to regrow lost teeth, much like sharks and alligators. The conservation of odontogenic gene networks across species suggests that the blueprint for tooth renewal still exists within us—waiting to be reawakened by future discoveries.

Conclusion

The evolution of human teeth reflects a complex interplay of genetics, diet, and environmental adaptation. From early primates with simple, generalized dentition to modern humans with specialized teeth, changes in tooth structure and function have been driven by dietary shifts and lifestyle modifications. The transition from a predominantly herbivorous diet to an omnivorous one led to the development of stronger enamel, varied tooth morphology, and a reduction in jaw size. The advent of cooking and food processing further influenced dental evolution by reducing selective pressure for large, robust teeth.

Despite these evolutionary adaptations, modern human teeth still face challenges, including malocclusion, dental caries, and wear due to contemporary dietary habits. Understanding the evolutionary history of teeth provides insights into oral health, guiding better dental care and treatment approaches. By studying past adaptations, we can better anticipate future trends in human dentition and oral health needs.

Chapter:3

Teeth and Diet: Coevolution in Science

Long ago, in a dense prehistoric jungle, a curious little primate named **Lumo** clung to the branches of an ancient fig tree. His sharp eyes scanned the canopy for the ripest fruit. His tribe had always relied on their teeth—strong and broad, perfect for crushing nuts and tearing fibrous leaves. But today, something was different.

Lumo had discovered a strange, softer fruit—one that required less effort to chew. As he bit into it, the sweet pulp burst in his mouth, delighting his senses. He didn't know it yet, but this moment was a turning point in history.

As generations passed, those who feasted on softer fruits and cooked foods found their jaws changing, shrinking ever so slightly. Their teeth became smaller, more refined, adapting to this new way of eating. In return, the plants, too, evolved—producing sweeter, juicier fruits to attract hungry primates, ensuring their seeds were spread far and wide.

Teeth and diet had entered a silent pact, shaping each other in ways no creature could have foreseen. From the razor-sharp fangs of predators to the grinding molars of plant-eaters, from the crushing jaws of early humans to the neatly aligned teeth of modern civilization—every bite in history told a story of survival, adaptation, and change.

And so, with every smile we flash today, we carry a whisper of that ancient tale—a story of evolution written not in words, but in enamel and bone.

Evolution is the continuous and gradual development of inherited traits in living organisms across successive generations. This fundamental biological process results in genetic and phenotypic diversity at all levels of life. In the mid-nineteenth century, Charles Darwin proposed the theory of evolution through natural selection, explaining that organisms produce more offspring than can survive in their environment. Those with beneficial adaptations are more likely to thrive, reproduce, and pass on their advantageous traits to the next generation.

All living organisms on Earth are believed to have originated from a common ancestor, known as the Last Universal Common Ancestor (LUCA). The modern evolutionary synthesis, formulated in the early twentieth century, combined Darwin's natural selection theory with Mendelian genetics, providing a more comprehensive understanding of evolution through the discipline of population genetics. Evolution is now widely regarded as one of the most substantiated scientific theories, with extensive evidence from various disciplines, including biology, anthropology, psychology, astrophysics, chemistry, geology, physics, mathematics, behavioral sciences, and social sciences (Ashraf & Sarfraz, 2016; National Geographic Society, 2019).

Human Dentition: Structure and Function

In mammals, the primary function of dentition is to capture, break down, and process food, facilitated by the hardness of dental tissues and the distinct crown shapes of different tooth types. In humans, teeth also play a crucial role in speech articulation, phonetics, and facial aesthetics.

Human dentition is classified as heterodont and diphyodont. Heterodonty refers to the presence of different types of teeth, namely incisors, canines, premolars, and molars, each specialized for distinct functions. Diphyodonty means humans develop two sets of teeth throughout life: the primary dentition (deciduous or milk teeth) and the permanent dentition (adult teeth). The primary dentition consists of 20 teeth, while the permanent dentition includes 32 teeth, distributed across the maxilla (upper jaw) and mandible (lower jaw) (Hovorakova et al., 2018; Wang et al., 2019).

From an anthropological perspective, dentition plays a pivotal role in human evolution. Teeth are highly resistant to environmental factors, making them an essential subject in comparative and evolutionary population studies. Specific morphological traits in teeth exhibit population-based variations, aiding in ancestry determination. Features such as shovel-shaped incisors, Carabelli's cusp, hypocone formation, and peg-shaped lateral incisors serve as distinguishing markers of genetic lineage.

Additionally, dentition provides valuable insights into an individual's diet, habits, and occupational background. The degree of tooth wear, enamel attrition, and dental anomalies can offer clues about an individual's lifestyle and cultural practices (Kjær, 2014; Krishan et al., 2015; Christensen et al., 2019; Kurniawan et al., 2020a).

Dentition in Forensic Identification

Human dentition plays a vital role in forensic identification due to its uniqueness and resilience. No two individuals, including monozygotic (identical) twins, have identical dental structures. Key identifying characteristics include tooth morphology, shape, wear patterns, anomalies, color, and restoration history.

Unlike other biological tissues, teeth resist decomposition, high temperatures, and mechanical trauma, making them valuable for postmortem identification. Forensic odontologists, in collaboration with dental anthropologists and forensic pathologists, analyze dental evidence to determine sex, age, ancestry, bite mark patterns, and dental records comparisons in forensic investigations (Krishan et al., 2015; Kurniawan et al., 2020b).

Evolutionary Changes in Human Dentition

Nearly all vertebrate species possess teeth or denticle-like structures, but their morphology and attachment mechanisms vary. In non-mammalian vertebrates, teeth typically lack roots and are anchored to the jawbone through ankylosis or fibrous connections. In contrast, mammalian teeth are embedded in alveolar sockets and connected via the periodontal ligament, allowing for mobility and load distribution.

Humans share a common mammalian ancestor with species such as rodents, whose dental formula includes 6 incisors, 2 canines, 8 premolars, and 6 molars per arch (Jheon et al., 2013; Enault et al., 2018).

One of the most significant evolutionary changes in humans is the reduction in jaw size over time. This shift is largely attributed to dietary changes and language development. The transition from hunting and gathering to agriculture-based diets reduced the need for large, powerful jaws. The consumption of softer, processed foods further contributed to the reduction in jaw size. Additionally, the development of language and vocal articulation required a more flexible oral cavity, leading to mandibular shrinkage (Emes et al., 2011; Polanski, 2011).

Early hominins exhibited megadontia, characterized by enlarged molars and thick enamel, which facilitated the consumption of tough, fibrous vegetation. In contrast, the genus Homo evolved smaller molars, aided by the use of stone tools and cooking methods that softened food.

Another key difference is the reduction in sexual dimorphism of canines. Early hominin males had significantly larger canines, whereas in modern humans, canines are more uniform between sexes. Similarly, molar size distribution has shifted—while early hominins had the largest second molars, modern humans have the largest first molars (Emes et al., 2011; Guatelli-Steinberg, 2018).

In terms of enamel thickness, early hominins had thicker enamel layers, offering protection against abrasive diets(Ungar, 2012). Additionally, tooth calcification patterns in early hominins closely resembled those of non-human primates, reflecting their slower developmental growth rates (Smith, 2013).

Dental Microwear Analysis: Insights into Diet

Dental microwear analysis is a powerful tool for reconstructing dietary patterns in paleoanthropology. Microscopic wear marks on tooth surfaces provide clues about an individual's mastication process and food consistency.

2D analysis involves scanning electron microscopy (SEM), which allows high-resolution visualization of wear features. A standardized method includes cleaning the tooth surface, molding with polyvinyl siloxane, and casting with epoxy resin, followed by microscopic examination (Mihlbachler et al., 2012).

3D analysis utilizes optical profilometry and Scale-Sensitive Fractal Analysis (SSFA) to create high-resolution 3D models of wear patterns. Surface analysis is performed using ISO parameters and digital imaging software (DeSantis, 2016).

Dental microwear patterns vary according to chewing dynamics. Occlusal wear is divided into:

- Shearing facets – involved in slicing food.
- Grinding facets – involved in crushing food during the power stroke of mastication (Martínez et al., 2016; Alrousan et al., 2019).

Despite its accuracy, dental microwear analysis faces challenges, such as small sample sizes, which can limit the statistical reliability of studies. However, it remains an essential method for studying dietary habits and evolutionary adaptations (Ungar, 2012; DeSantis, 2016).

Tools for studying coevolution of diet and teeth

The study of the coevolution of diet and teeth requires a multidisciplinary approach that integrates fossil analysis, molecular biology, bioinformatics, and experimental studies. Teeth, being highly durable structures, preserve well in the fossil record and provide valuable insights into dietary adaptations over evolutionary time. Researchers use a combination of imaging technologies, chemical analysis, genetic tools, and ethnographic studies to reconstruct how diet has influenced dental morphology and function in different species, including humans.

Fossil and dental analysis tools are essential for studying physical evidence of evolutionary changes in teeth. Micro-CT scanning allows high-resolution imaging of fossilized teeth, helping researchers examine internal structures, enamel thickness, and developmental patterns. Stable isotope analysis is another powerful technique that identifies dietary habits based on the chemical composition of tooth enamel, providing clues about ancient diets. Dental microwear analysis studies the microscopic wear patterns on teeth to infer whether an organism consumed tough plant materials, meat, or processed foods. Similarly, 3D morphometric analysis, using software like Morphologika or Avizo, helps reconstruct changes in tooth shape across evolutionary timelines.

Advances in genetics and molecular biology have further expanded our understanding of the coevolution of diet and teeth. Ancient DNA (aDNA) sequencing extracts genetic material from teeth, revealing information about genetic adaptations to diet, such as lactose tolerance and amylase gene variations. Comparative genomics compares DNA sequences across species to identify mutations associated with specific dietary adaptations. Additionally, metagenomics investigates the evolution of the oral microbiome, shedding light on how dietary shifts, such as the transition to agriculture, have influenced oral health and disease patterns.

In addition to fossil and genetic studies, experimental and ethnographic approaches provide valuable real-world insights. Controlled feeding experiments help researchers understand how different foods affect tooth wear, decay, and development. Meanwhile, ethnographic studies focus on indigenous and hunter-gatherer populations to analyze their diets and dental health, offering comparisons to modern processed food diets. These studies highlight the impact of diet on oral health, including the rise of dental caries with the consumption of refined sugars.

The integration of bioinformatics and artificial intelligence (AI) has revolutionized evolutionary studies. Phylogenetic software like MEGA and BEAST allows researchers to reconstruct evolutionary trees of dental adaptations, showing how tooth morphology has evolved in response to dietary changes. Additionally, AI and machine learning models are increasingly being used to classify dental traits and predict dietary patterns based on fossilized remains.

By combining these diverse tools, researchers can construct a comprehensive understanding of how diet has shaped dental evolution over millions of years. This interdisciplinary approach provides critical insights into human health, evolutionary biology, and the future of dental adaptation in changing environmental and dietary landscapes.

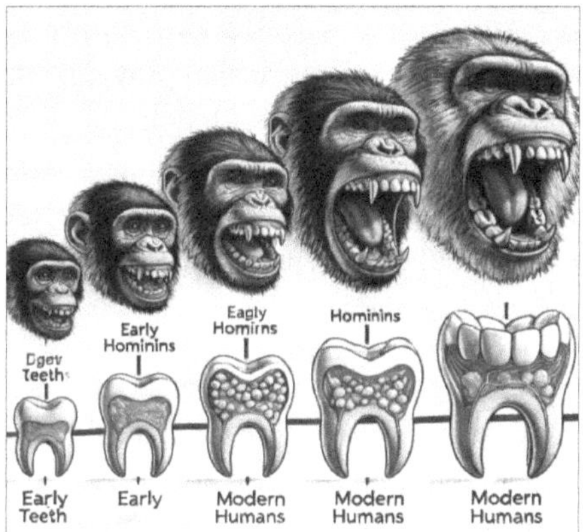

This image illustrating the evolutionary changes in human teeth over time, highlighting diet-related adaptations.

Lessons from Evolution for Today's Dietary Practices

The evolution of human diet has shaped not only our teeth but also our digestive system, metabolism, and overall health. By studying evolutionary adaptations, we can gain insights into how modern dietary habits impact health and how we can make better food choices. The shift from a hunter-gatherer diet to agriculture and then to processed food consumption has led to various health consequences. Understanding these evolutionary changes can help guide modern dietary practices for better health and longevity.

One of the key lessons from evolution is the importance of dietary diversity. Early humans had a varied diet that included fruits, vegetables, nuts, seeds, and lean protein from wild animals. This provided essential nutrients and helped maintain metabolic balance. In contrast, modern diets often rely heavily on processed foods, refined carbohydrates, and added sugars, leading to obesity, diabetes, and heart disease. Studies suggest that reintroducing a diverse range of whole foods, as seen in Paleolithic diets, can improve health outcomes by reducing inflammation and maintaining stable blood sugar levels.

Another crucial insight is the role of fiber-rich foods in gut health. Ancient diets were rich in fiber from plant-based sources, which supported a healthy gut microbiome. The modern shift to low-fiber diets has been linked to gut dysbiosis, leading to conditions such as irritable bowel syndrome (IBS), colorectal cancer, and metabolic disorders. Increasing fiber intake through fruits, vegetables, and whole grains can help restore gut microbiota balance and improve digestion.

The evolution of lactose and gluten tolerance also provides important dietary lessons. Lactose tolerance evolved in some human populations due to dairy farming, but many individuals still experience lactose intolerance. Similarly, while gluten consumption increased with the advent of agriculture, gluten sensitivity and celiac disease remain concerns. Recognizing individual genetic predispositions to food intolerances can help in making personalized dietary choices.

A significant evolutionary change has been the impact of cooking and food processing on digestion. Cooking made nutrients more bioavailable and reduced the energy required for digestion, allowing for brain expansion. However, excessive modern food processing has led to nutrient depletion and the prevalence of artificial additives, which contribute to metabolic disorders. Reducing ultra-processed food intake and focusing on natural, minimally processed foods can enhance nutrient absorption and metabolic health.

Lastly, evolution teaches us about intermittent fasting and energy balance. Early humans often experienced periods of feast and famine, which may have contributed to metabolic flexibility. Modern diets with constant access to food and excessive caloric intake have contributed to obesity and metabolic diseases. Research suggests that intermittent fasting or time-restricted eating can help regulate insulin levels, improve cardiovascular health, and promote longevity.

By applying these evolutionary dietary lessons—emphasizing whole foods, fiber, personalized nutrition, minimal processing, and intermittent fasting—we can align our modern diets with our biological adaptations and improve overall health.

Section 2:

Cultural and Social Implications of Smiles

Chapter 4:
Cultural Perspectives on Smiling

In a bustling marketplace in Kyoto, Japan, a young traveler named Emma wandered through the maze of lantern-lit streets. The scent of freshly grilled yakitori filled the air, blending with the quiet hum of the crowd. She was mesmerized but also lost, her map offering little help.

Spotting an elderly shopkeeper arranging ceramic teacups, Emma approached him with a hopeful smile and pointed at her phone, attempting to ask for directions. The man listened intently, his face calm, then responded—not with words, but with a small, closed-mouth smile and a polite nod.

Emma hesitated. In her hometown of New York, a smile was an open invitation—warm, friendly, and often followed by cheerful conversation. But here, the shopkeeper's reserved expression felt different, almost unreadable. Was he being polite? Was he amused by her confusion? Or was he simply unsure how to help?

Still, he motioned for her to follow. Quietly, they walked through the winding streets until he stopped at a crossroads, pointed in one direction, and gave another subtle smile before bowing and walking away.

Emma stood there, reflecting on the exchange. His smile had been restrained yet kind, distant yet sincere. She had always believed that a smile was universal, but now she saw it wasn't just about movement of the lips—it carried layers of meaning shaped by culture.

In some countries, like the United States or Brazil, smiles were given freely, even to strangers—a sign of warmth and approachability. But in Japan, a smile could be an expression of politeness rather than happiness, sometimes even used to mask discomfort. In Russia, people often smiled only when they truly meant it, not out of habit. In Thailand, the "Land of Smiles," different types of smiles conveyed everything from joy to apology.

This simple but profound moment in Kyoto changed how Emma saw the world. A smile was more than just a universal gesture—it was a reflection of history, traditions, and the unspoken language of every culture.

The story of Emma in Kyoto highlights how a smile, though seemingly universal, carries different meanings across cultures. A smile can communicate various emotions and intentions, such as happiness, affiliation, social status, or even subtle messages of politeness or discomfort. However, the interpretation of a smile depends on both the person smiling and the one perceiving it, with cultural background playing a crucial role in shaping these perceptions. Research suggests that the intensity of a smile further influences its interpretation—higher-intensity smiles are generally perceived as more positive and authentic, while lower-intensity smiles may sometimes be seen as polite or even masking negative emotions. Studies on Chinese smiles, for instance, reveal that stronger smiles are interpreted as more positive and genuine, reinforcing the idea that both cultural norms and expression intensity shape how we understand this simple yet complex facial gesture. Emma's experience in Japan is a perfect example of this—what she initially saw as a reserved or distant smile was, in fact, an expression of politeness rooted in cultural tradition

Smiling is widely regarded as a positive social behavior. As Louis Armstrong famously sang, *"When you smile, the world smiles with you."* Many self-help books and communication experts encourage smiling, as it is believed to improve interpersonal interactions. These common beliefs are supported by research, which has consistently shown that people who smile are perceived as happier (Otta et al., 1994), more attractive, sociable, and competent (Hess et al., 2002; Matsumoto & Kudoh, 1993). Smiling individuals are also seen as more likable (Palmer & Simmons, 1995), approachable, and friendly, often creating an expectation of a positive and secure interaction (Miles, 2009).

A Diplomatic Smile Mishap

During an international business meeting between American and Russian executives, a misunderstanding arose due to different cultural interpretations of a smile. The American team, following their cultural norm, frequently smiled throughout discussions to create a friendly atmosphere and signal goodwill. However, their Russian counterparts viewed these constant smiles as insincere or even suspicious—after all, in Russia, excessive smiling, especially in formal settings, can be interpreted as a sign of dishonesty or hidden motives. The tension was finally resolved when a cultural consultant stepped in to explain the differing expectations surrounding smiling in each culture. This situation illustrates how smiles, though universal, do not always carry the same meaning across cultures.

Culture and the Science of Smiling

Cultural differences play a significant role in shaping social behaviors, including how nonverbal cues like smiling are interpreted (Matsumoto, 2006; Leung & Cohen, 2011). Psychological research over the past few decades has increasingly focused on non-WEIRD (Western, Educated, Industrialized, Rich, and Democratic) societies, highlighting that findings from Western psychological studies may not always apply across different cultures (Smith et al., 2013). While cross-cultural psychology is a growing field, the way smiles are socially perceived across diverse cultural contexts remains relatively underexplored. For example, many studies have compared Eastern and Western cultural attitudes toward smiling, but there is a lack of research beyond this binary comparison (Hess et al., 2000).

A study by Rychlowska et al. (2015) explored this gap by investigating how cultural homogeneity or heterogeneity influences attitudes toward smiling. In more diverse societies, where populations have historically migrated from multiple origins, smiles are more likely to be used as affiliative signals to build trust among strangers. In contrast, in culturally homogenous societies, smiling may be interpreted differently, sometimes even as a sign of lower social status or submission. For instance, in Japan—a relatively homogenous society—people may smile to mask negative emotions or discomfort, rather than to express happiness. In contrast, in the United States—a highly diverse nation—smiles are more commonly used as genuine social engagement tools.

The Many Meanings of a Smile

Smiles are not a one-size-fits-all expression; they convey a variety of psychological and social signals. They can indicate positive emotions, social intentions, or even social dominance (Matsumoto & Willingham, 2009). Over time, researchers have proposed different ways to classify smiles. One of the earliest distinctions, made by Duchenne (1862), separates *Duchenne smiles*—genuine smiles that engage both the mouth and eye muscles—from *non-Duchenne smiles*, which involve only the mouth and are often perceived as insincere. However, recent research suggests that the Duchenne marker is not universally recognized across cultures (Abe et al., 2002; Thibault et al., 2012).

To better understand the role of smiles in social interactions, Niedenthal et al. (2010) proposed the Simulation of Smiles Model, which classifies smiles based on their function rather than physical features.

This model identifies three primary types of smiles:

1. **Enjoyment Smiles** – These smiles occur spontaneously in moments of genuine pleasure or success. For example, when a child receives a surprise birthday gift, their wide-eyed, full-faced smile reflects pure joy.

2. **Affiliative Smiles** – These smiles serve to build social bonds and communicate goodwill. A store clerk's warm smile when greeting a customer, or a new neighbor's friendly grin, helps to establish a sense of trust and connection. Unlike enjoyment smiles, affiliative smiles do not necessarily stem from personal happiness but serve a social function.

3. **Dominance Smiles** – These smiles communicate social status or control. They can appear as smug, condescending, or even threatening, depending on the context. A coach smirking confidently after their team wins a match or a high-status executive subtly smiling while making a decisive statement in a boardroom are examples of dominance smiles.

Chang & Vermeulen (2010) argue that enjoyment and affiliative smiles often look alike, making it difficult to differentiate them based on physical features alone—context plays a crucial role in understanding their meaning. Rychlowska et al. (2015) further demonstrated that cultural diversity influences the way people perceive these different types of smiles. In societies with high cultural heterogeneity (such as the United States or Canada), affiliative smiles are more commonly endorsed as a way to foster cooperation in diverse communities. In contrast, in culturally homogenous societies (such as Japan or Finland), dominance smiles may be more prevalent as they align with hierarchical social structures.

Ultimately, while smiling is a universal human expression, its meaning and social function vary significantly across cultures. A smile can be a bridge between strangers, a signal of power, or even a way to hide discomfort. Understanding these nuances is crucial for effective cross-cultural communication, particularly in a world where globalization and migration continue to shape social interactions. So next time someone smiles at you, take a moment to consider—what story might their smile be telling?

The Role of Facial Expressions in Communicating Emotional Intensity

The ability to convey emotional intensity through facial expressions plays a crucial ecological role, as it provides valuable clues about an individual's potential behavior. In many species, intense signals of aggression often precede an actual attack—if the recipient of such signals does not retreat, a physical confrontation may follow. This principle also applies to humans, who frequently rely on facial expressions to communicate emotions and their intensity. However, the exact mechanisms behind this complex form of nonverbal communication remain unclear.

To better understand how humans interpret facial expressions, researchers conducted a perception-based, data-driven study to mathematically model how individuals in two distinct cultures—East Asian and Western European—classify six fundamental emotions: happiness, surprise, fear, disgust, anger, and sadness. The study involved 120 participants who evaluated these emotions and their intensity based on facial movements. The findings revealed that people expect facial expressions to follow a structured, dynamic signaling pattern over time, where specific facial movements convey both the type of emotion (emotion classifiers) and its intensity (emotion intensifiers).

How Facial Expressions Convey Emotion and Intensity

The study found that emotional expressions follow a multi-component compositional signaling structure, meaning different facial movements contribute separately to identifying the emotion and gauging its intensity. Notably:

1. Emotion classifiers—the facial movements that define the emotion itself—tend to be distinct across emotions.
2. Emotion intensifiers, which indicate the strength of an emotion, often peak at different times than classifiers and are communicated through variations in movement amplitude (e.g., a bigger smile or a more furrowed brow).
3. Emotion intensifiers are more similar across different emotions, while classifiers remain highly specific. This suggests that facial expressions use a broad-plus-specific signaling structure, where some elements of expression (like widening the eyes) are shared across emotions, while others (like a smirk versus a scowl) differentiate between them.

Cross-Cultural Differences in Emotional Interpretation

The study also explored how individuals from different cultural backgrounds interpret emotional intensity in facial expressions. While East Asian and Western European participants showed similar expectations for high-intensity expressions of threat-related emotions—such as anger, fear, and disgust—they differed in their interpretations of low-intensity expressions for non-threatening emotions, such as happiness and sadness.

For instance, in many Western cultures, happiness is often expressed with broad smiles that show teeth, while in East Asian cultures, more subtle or closed-mouth smiles are commonly used, especially in formal or social settings. Similarly, sadness may be displayed with distinct facial cues in different cultural contexts, influencing how it is perceived by observers from different backgrounds. These differences highlight how cultural norms shape emotional communication and could impact cross-cultural interactions.

This study provides new insights into the intricate ways in which facial expressions convey complex emotional signals. The findings suggest that facial expressions are not static but dynamic systems that communicate both emotion type and intensity through distinct yet interconnected facial movements. Understanding these mechanisms not only enhances our knowledge of human communication but also has practical implications for fields such as psychology, artificial intelligence, and cross-cultural communication.

In essence, our faces do more than just reflect emotions—they serve as sophisticated communication tools that convey a wealth of information, shaping our interactions in ways we may not even consciously recognize.

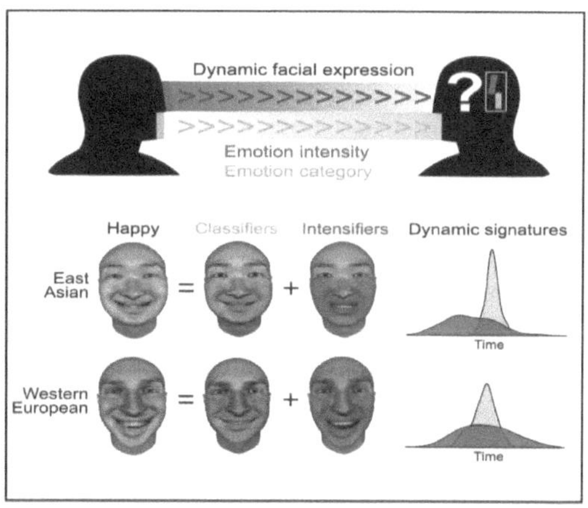

Figure depicting the Role of Facial Expressions in Communicating Emotional Intensity

The Historical Evolution of the Meaning of a Smile

A smile is one of the most universally recognized facial expressions, yet its meaning has shifted significantly throughout history. While today a smile is commonly associated with happiness, friendliness, and warmth, its interpretation has varied across different cultures, historical periods, and social contexts. From the restrained smiles of the Renaissance to the confident grins of the modern world, the meaning of a smile has reflected societal values, artistic representations, and cultural norms.

Smiling in Ancient Civilizations: Symbol of Power and Mystery

In ancient civilizations, smiles were often rare in artistic and social depictions. In Ancient Egypt, for example, figures in sculptures and paintings were typically portrayed with calm, stoic expressions, as these were associated with wisdom and dignity. A broad smile was not seen as a sign of joy but could indicate foolishness or even madness. Similarly, in Ancient Greece, philosophers and intellectuals were typically depicted with serious expressions, reflecting the cultural belief that reason and self-control were more important than overt emotional displays. However, smiles were sometimes used in theatrical performances to signal different emotional states, showing that their meaning was already complex and context-dependent.

The Romans, on the other hand, recognized the strategic use of smiles in social and political life. While elite Romans were often portrayed with serious, authoritative expressions in statues, historical accounts suggest that smiling could be used as a tool for persuasion, diplomacy, and even deception. Julius Caesar and other leaders were known for their ability to use a smile to disarm opponents and win public favor.

The Middle Ages: The Smile of the Fool and the Sinful

During the medieval period, particularly in Europe, smiling was often associated with negative qualities. The Church emphasized solemnity and spiritual devotion, and excessive smiling or laughter was sometimes linked to sinfulness, moral weakness, or a lack of seriousness. In medieval art, saints and religious figures were typically portrayed with calm, composed expressions, reinforcing the idea that holiness required restraint.

However, smiling was sometimes depicted in negative contexts, such as in the case of the "Laughing Fool" motif. Court jesters and trickster figures were often shown grinning widely, symbolizing their role as outsiders who mocked authority and disrupted social norms. Smiling, in this sense, was linked to deception, folly, or even heresy, as unrestrained laughter was sometimes viewed as a sign of demonic possession or lack of divine grace.

The Renaissance: A New Appreciation for the Subtle Smile

The Renaissance period (14th–17th century) marked a turning point in the representation of smiles, particularly in art. This era, which celebrated humanism and the rediscovery of classical ideals, introduced a more nuanced approach to facial expressions. Perhaps the most famous example is Leonardo da Vinci's Mona Lisa, whose enigmatic smile has fascinated viewers for centuries. Unlike the broad, exaggerated smiles seen in later periods, Renaissance smiles were often subtle, reflecting an intellectual or mysterious quality rather than mere happiness.

This shift also reflected broader cultural changes. As Renaissance thinkers emphasized individuality and personal expression, smiling began to be associated with intelligence, charm, and emotional depth. However, broad, open-mouthed smiles were still rare in formal portraits, as they were considered inappropriate for the upper classes, who valued restraint and composure.

The 18th and 19th Centuries: The Social Smile and Changing Etiquette

By the 18th century, the Enlightenment brought a greater appreciation for emotions, including joy and laughter. Smiling became more acceptable in social interactions, particularly among the emerging middle class. Portraits from this period occasionally featured more relaxed expressions, though full smiles with visible teeth remained uncommon, partly due to dental hygiene concerns.

In the 19th century, with the rise of photography, a strange paradox occurred: while smiling became more common in everyday life, it was largely absent in early photographs. Long exposure times meant that subjects had to hold their expressions for extended periods, leading to the prevalence of serious, neutral expressions. Additionally, Victorian-era etiquette still associated wide smiles with lower social status, and many people viewed excessive grinning as undignified or improper. However, as dental care improved and advertising began to influence popular culture, the smile gradually became associated with beauty, health, and confidence.

The 20th Century: The Commercialization of the Smile

The 20th century saw an explosion in the prominence of the smile, particularly in Western culture. The rise of Hollywood, advertising, and consumer culture transformed the smile into a powerful symbol of success, friendliness, and approachability. Movie stars like Marilyn Monroe and Audrey Hepburn popularized the idea of the radiant, camera-ready smile, while advertisements for toothpaste, soft drinks, and beauty products reinforced the association between a bright smile and attractiveness.

The "smile revolution" was further fueled by advancements in photography and the development of instant cameras like the Polaroid, which encouraged people to smile naturally in photos. The phrase "Say cheese!" became common, reinforcing the expectation that smiling was the appropriate expression for photographs. This trend spread globally, though some cultures, particularly in East Asia, continued to maintain a more reserved approach to smiling in formal settings.

The 21st Century: The Smile in a Digital Age

Today, the meaning of a smile continues to evolve, influenced by technology and globalization. Social media platforms like Instagram, TikTok, and Facebook have made smiling an essential part of self-presentation, with people carefully curating images that project happiness and confidence. Emojis, including the ubiquitous 😊 and 😂, have added a new dimension to how smiles are used in digital communication, sometimes replacing or exaggerating real-life emotional expressions.

At the same time, cultural differences in smiling persist. While Western cultures generally encourage open, friendly smiles in both professional and casual settings, some East Asian cultures emphasize more reserved expressions, particularly in formal situations. Psychological research has also shown that the meaning of a smile can vary based on context—while a smile may indicate happiness or friendliness, it can also convey sarcasm, embarrassment, or even dominance.

From its historical associations with power, folly, and mystery to its modern role as a symbol of joy and social connection, the smile has undergone significant transformations over time. While its basic function as an expression of emotion remains constant, cultural norms, artistic trends, and social expectations have all shaped how smiles are perceived and used.

As societies continue to evolve, so too will the meaning of the smile. Whether in face-to-face interactions, art, or digital communication, the smile remains a powerful, adaptable expression—one that speaks volumes about the values and emotions of the people who wear it.

Now let us dive deeper into cultural aspects of smile by some case studies:

The meaning of a smile has changed significantly throughout history, influenced by cultural norms, technological advancements, and social expectations. From the reserved expressions of the Renaissance to the digital smiles of today, the interpretation of a smile varies depending on time, place, and context. The following case studies illustrate how the perception and significance of a smile have evolved over different periods and societies.

Case Study 1: The Mona Lisa's Enigmatic Smile (16th Century)

Historical Context:

Leonardo da Vinci's *Mona Lisa* (1503–1506) is one of the most analyzed artworks in history. The portrait depicts a woman, Lisa Gherardini, with a subtle and mysterious smile, a defining feature that has intrigued scholars, artists, and the public for centuries.

Analysis of the Smile:

During the Renaissance, expressions in portraiture were typically serious. Openly smiling faces were considered inappropriate, as they were associated with commoners, jesters, or even foolishness. The Mona Lisa's smile was a departure from the rigid expressions seen in most portraits of the time.

Da Vinci achieved this enigmatic effect through a technique called sfumato, which blended colors and shadows to create depth. This gave her smile an ambiguous quality—appearing cheerful from one angle and neutral from another.

Theories on the Meaning of the Smile:

- Some art historians believe her smile represents the Renaissance ideal of inner wisdom and self-restraint, aligning with the era's emphasis on balance and intellect.
- Others suggest that it reflects emotional depth, hinting at a secret or personal experience unknown to the viewer.
- Modern psychological research has examined how different observers perceive her smile based on lighting, mood, and angle, emphasizing how a single expression can have multiple interpretations.

Impact on Perception of Smiles:

The Mona Lisa's smile challenged the conventions of the time and paved the way for a more nuanced understanding of facial expressions in art. Today, her smile continues to captivate audiences, demonstrating how a simple facial gesture can evoke endless speculation and interpretation.

Case Study 2: Victorian-Era Photography and the "Unsuitable" Smile (19th Century)

Historical Context:

By the 19th century, photography had become more widely accessible. However, most portraits from this era depict people with serious and solemn expressions. The rarity of smiles in these images has often led modern viewers to mistakenly assume that people of the past were generally unhappy.

Reasons for the Lack of Smiling in Early Photographs:

1. Technical Limitations:
   - Early cameras required long exposure times (often several minutes), making it difficult to hold a smile without appearing unnatural or blurred.
   - A neutral or serious expression was easier to maintain during extended exposures.
2. Cultural Norms and Class Perception:
   - Smiling was often associated with lower social classes, drunkenness, or immaturity.
   - A restrained expression reflected Victorian values of dignity, self-control, and sophistication.
3. Dental Health Concerns:
   - Before modern dentistry, many people had poor dental health, making them reluctant to showcase their teeth in portraits.
   - Wealthier individuals, who could afford photography, may have preferred a closed-mouth expression to hide dental imperfections.

Notable Examples:

- Abraham Lincoln's photographs depict him with a stern and composed expression, reinforcing the idea that leaders should appear serious and authoritative.
- In contrast, rare images of people smiling from this era (such as the 1853 photograph of a laughing bayonet instructor) are notable exceptions that highlight how smiles were generally seen as unconventional in formal settings.

Shift in Attitudes Toward Smiling:

By the late 19th century, as photographic techniques improved and exposure times shortened, more natural expressions—including smiles—began appearing in casual and family portraits. However, formal portraits retained their seriousness well into the early 20th century.

Case Study 3: The Rise of Hollywood's "Perfect Smile" (20th Century)

Historical Context:

The 20th century marked a dramatic shift in how smiles were perceived, largely due to the influence of Hollywood and mass media. Smiling became a symbol of beauty, charm, and success, especially in Western societies.

Hollywood's Influence on Smiling Norms:

1. Celebrity Culture and the "Hollywood Smile":
    - Classic Hollywood icons such as Marilyn Monroe, Clark Gable, and Audrey Hepburn were known for their radiant smiles.
    - Their wide, white-toothed smiles set a new beauty standard, reinforcing the idea that smiling signified confidence and charisma.
2. The Role of Dentistry:
    - Advances in orthodontics and cosmetic dentistry in the 1930s and beyond made straight, white teeth more accessible.
    - Dental brands like Colgate and Crest began marketing oral hygiene as essential to achieving a "perfect" smile.

3. Advertising and Consumerism:
   - Companies used smiling models in advertisements to sell products, linking smiles to happiness, health, and desirability.
   - Brands like Coca-Cola popularized the idea that smiling (often while holding a soda) was a universal expression of joy and social connection.

Cultural Implications:

This period cemented the idea that smiling was not just a natural expression but an expectation, especially in media, advertising, and customer service industries.

Case Study 4: Cross-Cultural Differences – The American vs. Japanese Smile

Cultural Differences in Smiling:

While Western cultures, particularly the United States, emphasize frequent and open smiling as a sign of friendliness, some cultures interpret smiling differently.

1. The American Smile (Western Culture):
   - In the U.S., smiling is encouraged in social and professional settings.
   - Smiling conveys friendliness, confidence, and approachability, and is often expected even in customer service roles.
   - A broad smile is seen as a sign of trustworthiness and positive energy.
2. The Japanese Smile (East Asian Culture):
   - In Japan, smiling is sometimes used to mask discomfort, embarrassment, or politeness rather than genuine happiness.
   - A study by Rychlowska et al. (2015) found that homogeneous cultures (like Japan) tend to rely more on contextual cues to interpret emotions rather than facial expressions alone.
   - In formal business settings, excessive smiling may be perceived as unprofessional or insincere.

Real-World Implications:

These cultural differences can impact cross-cultural communication, leading to misunderstandings. For example, an American may interpret a Japanese person's reserved smile as coldness, while a Japanese person may see an American's enthusiastic smile as overly familiar.

Case Study 5: The Digital Smile – Emojis and Social Media (21st Century)

The Role of Technology in Changing Smiling Norms:

With the rise of texting and social media, digital smiles in the form of emojis have become an essential part of modern communication.

Key Changes in Smiling Behavior:

1. Emojis as a Substitute for Facial Expressions:
   - People now use 😊, 😂, and 😁 to convey emotions that might not be apparent in text-based conversations.
   - Emojis help prevent misinterpretation of messages by adding emotional context.
2. Different Cultural Interpretations of Emoji Smiles:
   - In Western cultures, 😂 (laughing face with tears) is often used to indicate amusement.
   - In East Asian cultures, 😊 (smiling face) is more commonly used to maintain social harmony rather than express genuine joy.
3. The Rise of the "Social Media Smile":
   - Instagram and TikTok influencers frequently post images with bright, perfected smiles, reinforcing unrealistic beauty and happiness standards.
   - The pressure to appear happy online has contributed to the phenomenon of “fake smiling” for social validation.

Chapter 5:

Psychology of smiling

A smile is one of the simplest, yet most profound, human expressions. It requires no words, no grand gestures—just a slight movement of the lips, a gentle lift of the cheeks. And yet, it has the power to comfort, connect, and even transform lives. Psychologists have long studied the impact of smiling, uncovering its deep influence on emotions, social interactions, and even the brain's chemistry. But long before science explained it, people instinctively knew its magic. In a small town tucked between rolling green hills, one silent man proved just how powerful a single smile could be.

In a small town nestled between rolling green hills, there was a man named Elias. He was neither famous nor particularly remarkable—just an ordinary man with an unusual habit: he never spoke. Not because he couldn't, but because he chose not to.

Elias had arrived in town years ago, his past a mystery, and though people were curious, they eventually stopped asking questions. He lived a simple life, tending to his garden, helping elderly neighbors, and walking through the bustling town square every morning.

But despite his silence, Elias had an extraordinary ability—he could make people feel seen. How? With a smile.

It was not the polite, fleeting smile exchanged between strangers, nor the rehearsed grin of customer service. His was different—genuine, warm, and deeply present. When he smiled at someone, it was as if, for that moment, they mattered in a way they had forgotten they did.

The weary baker, exhausted from kneading dough before dawn, found his spirits lifted when Elias nodded at him with that quiet acknowledgment. The lonely widow who sat by her window every afternoon, lost in memories, felt comforted when Elias passed by and smiled. The mischievous children, often scolded for their pranks, felt understood when he gave them a knowing smirk.

No one could explain it, but something about Elias's silent kindness was contagious. Slowly, the town began to change. Strangers exchanged smiles more often, conversations felt lighter, and even those who had little to say found solace in shared moments of warmth.

One day, a traveler passing through asked an old shopkeeper, "Who is that man? Why does everyone here seem to know him?"

The shopkeeper chuckled. "That's Elias. He doesn't say much, but he taught us something priceless—sometimes, a smile speaks louder than words."

And just like that, Elias's quiet legacy continued, proving what psychologists have long studied: that a smile is not just an expression, but a force capable of transforming human connection, one silent moment at a time.

The story of Elias illustrates a profound psychological truth: smiles have a transformative impact on human connection and well-being. Although he never spoke, Elias's ability to convey warmth and understanding through his smile changed the emotional landscape of an entire town. His silent yet powerful interactions reflect what psychologists have long studied—the psychological and social effects of smiling.

The Science Behind a Smile

Smiling is more than a simple facial expression; it is a fundamental aspect of human communication. Research in psychology and neuroscience suggests that smiling activates the brain's reward system. When Elias smiled at townspeople, their brains likely responded by releasing neurotransmitters such as dopamine, serotonin, and endorphins, which are associated with happiness and reduced stress (Hennenlotter et al., 2005). This neurological reaction explains why the baker felt uplifted despite his exhaustion and why the widow found comfort in Elias's presence.

Furthermore, the mere act of smiling can improve mood through the facial feedback hypothesis. According to this theory, the physical act of smiling sends signals to the brain that reinforce positive emotions (Strack, Martin, & Stepper, 1988). Elias's genuine smile likely triggered this response in those who received it, creating a ripple effect of positivity in the town.

Social Bonding and Emotional Contagion

Elias's silent interactions demonstrate the concept of emotional contagion—the phenomenon where emotions are transferred between individuals through nonverbal cues (Hatfield, Cacioppo, & Rapson, 1994). When people observed Elias's genuine smile, they unconsciously mirrored it, leading to an increase in their own positive emotions. This explains why the town gradually became warmer and more connected.

Additionally, smiles serve as social signals that foster trust and cooperation. Studies have shown that people who smile are perceived as more approachable, competent, and trustworthy (Mehu, Little, & Dunbar, 2007). Elias's ability to make people feel "seen" likely stemmed from his nonverbal communication, which conveyed empathy and recognition.

Psychological Implications of Silent Kindness

Elias's decision to remain silent yet express kindness through smiling also highlights the importance of nonverbal communication in social interactions. In psychological research, nonverbal cues often carry more weight than words in conveying emotions (Mehrabian, 1972). Elias's silent presence, accompanied by his authentic smile, created a unique form of social bonding that required no verbal confirmation.

Moreover, his ability to uplift others aligns with positive psychology principles. Acts of kindness, even as simple as a smile, contribute to an overall sense of well-being and social harmony (Lyubomirsky, King, & Diener, 2005). Elias's influence in the town exemplifies how small, consistent gestures can cultivate an environment of mutual care and understanding.

Elias's story is a testament to the psychological power of a smile. His quiet legacy illustrates how smiles can uplift individuals, strengthen communities, and transform human interactions. Psychological research supports this phenomenon, demonstrating that smiling is not merely an expression but a force that fosters connection, trust, and emotional well-being. In essence, Elias proved that sometimes, a smile speaks louder than words.

Let us understand the psychological effect of smile via one more anecdote.

In a quiet city, where life rushed by in hurried footsteps and busy schedules, lived a woman named Maya. She was known for her kindness, her diligence at work, and her quiet presence. But there was one thing Maya was never known for—her smile.

It wasn't that she was unhappy. She felt joy like everyone else, found humor in everyday moments, and cherished the warmth of friends and family. But she had spent years perfecting the art of smiling without showing her teeth. It was a habit formed in childhood, when a classmate had pointed at her slightly misaligned teeth and laughed. The teasing had been brief, but the memory lasted. Since then, Maya had trained herself to hide her smile behind closed lips or a strategically placed hand.

She became an expert at avoiding photos, ducking compliments, and suppressing laughter when it felt too unguarded. Over time, she convinced herself that it didn't matter—after all, she was smart, hardworking, and surrounded by people who cared about her. Why should a smile make any difference?

One evening, at a family gathering, her younger cousin giggled and said, "Maya, why do you never smile with your teeth?" The question was innocent, but it struck her in a way she didn't expect. Later that night, she stood in front of the mirror, forcing herself to smile naturally, fully. It had been so long since she had seen her own reflection like this. And for the first time, she wondered—had she been holding back more than just a smile?

The next morning, she made an impulsive decision. She booked an appointment with a dentist. Not because she wanted to chase some impossible standard of beauty, but because she wanted to feel free. Over the next few months, small changes began to take place. A minor orthodontic adjustment. A little whitening. A growing sense of confidence.

But the real transformation wasn't in her teeth—it was in her mind. She started smiling more, first hesitantly, then naturally. And with that came something she never anticipated: warmth from strangers, easier conversations, a lightness in social interactions. Her world hadn't changed, but somehow, it felt different. She realized she had spent years believing that her teeth were a flaw to be hidden when, in reality, they were simply a part of her.

Maya's story is not unique. Across the world, millions of people suppress their smiles, conscious of how their teeth might be perceived. But science and psychology both reveal that a smile is more than an expression—it shapes how we feel, how others respond to us, and even how we see ourselves. The connection between psychology and teeth is deeper than we often acknowledge, and understanding it can help us embrace the simple yet powerful act of smiling freely.

A smile is a powerful tool for human connection, influencing perceptions of warmth, trustworthiness, and attractiveness. However, the role of teeth in shaping a smile's psychological impact is often overlooked. Teeth contribute not only to aesthetics but also to self-esteem, social confidence, and overall emotional well-being (Niedenthal, 2007). Research suggests that individuals with well-aligned, healthy teeth are perceived as more socially competent and approachable, while dental imperfections can lead to self-consciousness and reduced smiling behavior (Kershaw et al., 2008).

Facial expressions, particularly smiles, play a crucial role in emotional regulation and social interactions. The **facial feedback hypothesis** posits that smiling can induce positive emotions, even when the expression is forced (Soussignan, 2002). However, people with dental concerns often suppress their smiles, leading to a negative cycle where the lack of smiling reinforces feelings of insecurity and anxiety (Klages et al., 2004). In social situations, individuals with visible dental issues report higher levels of self-consciousness, affecting their willingness to engage in conversations and form relationships (Pithon et al., 2014).

The psychological impact of dental aesthetics is evident across different cultures. In Western societies, straight, white teeth are associated with health, success, and good hygiene, making them an unspoken social expectation (Shulman & Brehm, 2008). Conversely, in some indigenous communities, natural dental variations or deliberate modifications, such as tooth sharpening, hold cultural significance (Newton et al., 2003). Despite these differences, the universal human preference for symmetry and proportion in facial features suggests that dental alignment and appearance influence social desirability across populations (Samorodnitzky-Naveh et al., 2010).

Dental issues, particularly malocclusions, discoloration, or missing teeth, are linked to psychological distress and lower self-esteem (Dumitrescu et al., 2009). Adolescents with misaligned teeth often experience bullying and social exclusion, leading to long-term emotional effects (Agou et al., 2011). Adults, too, may feel embarrassed about their dental condition, impacting their confidence in professional and personal interactions (Phillips et al., 1997). Studies indicate that individuals seeking orthodontic or cosmetic dental treatments report significant improvements in self-image and psychological well-being post-treatment (Afroz et al., 2013).

Beyond aesthetics, oral health contributes to mental health in more direct ways. Chronic dental pain, often caused by untreated cavities or gum disease, can lead to irritability, stress, and even depressive symptoms (Gerritsen et al., 2010). Poor oral hygiene is also linked to systemic conditions, such as cardiovascular disease and diabetes, which can further affect mental health through the stress of managing chronic illness (Coachman et al., 2017).

With advancements in dental technology, treatments such as clear aligners, veneers, and digital smile design have made it easier to achieve an aesthetically pleasing smile. These interventions not only enhance appearance but also restore confidence, reinforcing the connection between oral health and psychological well-being (Pithon et al., 2014). Future research may continue to explore how dental interventions shape self-perception and social behavior, further highlighting the importance of a healthy, confident smile in psychological and emotional resilience.

Chapter 6:
Ancient Dental practices across cultures

Imagine a world where a toothache could mean a visit to the village shaman, who might chant over your head, extract the tooth with a sharpened rock, or even drill into it with a bow-powered tool—without anesthesia. In this world, teeth weren't just for chewing; they were symbols of power, status, and even spiritual significance.
The first dentist didn't wear a white coat. He didn't have a sterile clinic, nor did he wield a sleek, high-speed drill. Instead, he sat under the open sky, armed with sharpened flint, grinding away at an aching tooth while his patient clenched a wooden stick between trembling hands. This was over 9,000 years ago—long before the birth of modern medicine—when dental care was as much about survival as it was about tradition.

Across the sands of ancient Egypt, priests and healers mixed honey with crushed myrrh to soothe inflamed gums, while master artisans in the Mayan civilization meticulously inlaid jade and turquoise into teeth, transforming smiles into works of art. In Rome, wealthy citizens rinsed their mouths with imported urine, believing its ammonia cleansed their teeth—a practice that, surprisingly, wasn't entirely misguided.

But ancient dentistry was not just about remedies; it was a reflection of culture, power, and belief. For some, teeth were markers of status, adorned with gold or filed into intricate patterns. For others, they were sacred—carved, dyed, or extracted as offerings to the gods. The story of early dental practices is not just one of crude tools and curious traditions; it is the story of human ingenuity, resilience, and an enduring obsession with the perfect smile.

Traditional Healing Practices in India

The Indian subcontinent has been a hub of human migration since prehistoric times, as evidenced by archaeological discoveries and modern genetic studies. Even the earliest settlers possessed a profound understanding of the medicinal properties of plants and natural substances, utilizing them for therapeutic purposes. The vast repository of medical knowledge that has been passed down through generations is the result of centuries of trial and error, along with the exchange of healing practices among diverse communities and regions.

Over time, as scientific awareness has increased, traditional medicine has been required to align itself with the principles of modern biomedicine. The growing recognition of the intrinsic value of ancient healing practices has led to their integration into contemporary healthcare. As a result, India's major traditional medical systems—Ayurveda, Unani, and Siddha—have entered the mainstream, complementing biomedicine to create a more holistic approach to patient care. The challenge now lies in harmonizing these different medical traditions to address the healthcare needs of modern society effectively.

Ancient Medical Interventions in India

Archaeological excavations indicate that medical procedures, including dentistry and trepanation (the drilling or scraping of the skull to relieve pressure), were performed as early as 7000 BCE in the Indian subcontinent. The highly organized agricultural practices of the Indus Valley Civilization and their cultivation of medicinal plants suggest an advanced awareness of health and disease management. Additionally, their emphasis on hygiene, water sanitation, and urban planning further reflects their deep understanding of public health principles.

Unconventional Approaches to Dentistry

Unconventional medicine (UM) has been an integral part of human civilization since recorded history. Some of these practices, rooted in religious and cultural traditions, have been passed down through generations and remain in use today. While some unconventional methods are based on traditional wisdom and spiritual beliefs, others are regarded with skepticism due to their unverified nature. In ancient civilizations, these healing methods were typically performed by skilled practitioners, such as shamans, sages, or wise men, who were regarded as custodians of medical knowledge.

In contrast, modern dentistry is a highly regulated and science-driven healthcare profession that caters to an increasingly well-informed population. However, contemporary dental practice now faces challenges from various alternative and complementary health approaches. While some of these unconventional methods hold merit and have been scientifically validated, others lack empirical evidence and may even be misleading. The term "unconventional" is thus more appropriate than "alternative," as it encompasses both evidence-based and non-scientific practices that exist outside conventional healthcare.

The Use of Herbal Medicine in Dentistry

The term "medicinal plant" is not a botanical classification but rather a reference to the therapeutic properties of certain plant species. Despite significant advancements in medical science, plant-based medicine continues to play a crucial role in healthcare worldwide. The increasing awareness of the side effects and complications associated with synthetic drugs has led to a renewed interest in herbal medicine. Today, approximately 25% of pharmaceutical drugs are derived from plant sources, while many others are modeled after naturally occurring plant compounds.

Over the past few decades, extensive research has been conducted on the use of medicinal plants for treating various ailments. The commercial utilization and exploitation of herbal medicines have surged, as documented by several scholars. While much research has focused on the broader applications of medicinal plants, relatively few studies have specifically examined their role in treating oral and dental conditions.

Some studies have highlighted the use of medicinal plants in treating oral diseases. For instance, Sadangi et al. documented ten species of medicinal plants used by the tribal communities of Kalahandi district for treating ear and mouth disorders. Similarly, Jadhav identified 15 plant species traditionally used for managing different types of fever, while Kadel and Jain reported the use of 34 plant species for treating snakebites in the states of Madhya Pradesh and Chhattisgarh.

Traditional Herbal Remedies for Dental Care

Teeth are not only essential for chewing and digestion but also play a crucial role in speech and overall health. Poor oral hygiene, excessive consumption of sugary foods, and dietary imbalances can lead to various dental issues such as tooth decay, gum disease, and infections. Throughout history, people have relied on medicinal plants to maintain oral health and treat dental ailments.

Several researchers have explored the role of traditional medicine in dental care. Singh and Dhakre documented the use of Argemone mexicana, Azadirachta indica (neem), and Ocimum basilicum (basil) for promoting oral hygiene and treating dental problems. Arya and Prakash reported the use of Hedychium spicatum and Zanthoxylum armatum in traditional dental care practices. Acharya et al. identified 26 different herbal medicines used for treating dental diseases, while Kanwar et al. recorded the use of Achyranthes aspera, Aegle marmelos (bael), and Vitex negundo in oral healthcare among the locals of Kangra district. Additionally, Tomar's research in Meerut district highlighted the use of six plant species for treating dental caries, and Sharma and Joshi documented 30 medicinal plant species used in Almora district, with five specifically applied in dental care.

The integration of these herbal remedies into modern dental practices presents an opportunity to develop safer, more natural, and cost-effective treatments for oral health problems. However, scientific validation through rigorous clinical studies remains essential to ensure their efficacy and safety. As traditional and modern medicine continue to evolve together, the synergy between the two can provide more comprehensive healthcare solutions for future generations.

Traditional Oral Hygiene Practices in India

Traditional oral hygiene methods have been practiced for centuries, long before modern dentistry understood the role of dental plaque in oral health. Ancient hygiene techniques were not only aimed at cleansing the oral cavity but also at preventing and managing periodontal diseases, albeit without the scientific understanding we have today. Various natural remedies, including herbal products, chewing sticks, tongue cleaning, and mouth rinsing, were commonly used in Indian society to maintain oral health. Many of these methods have since been studied for their antibacterial, anti-inflammatory, and antioxidant properties, demonstrating their potential effectiveness in modern dental care.

Herbal Remedies for Oral Hygiene

Although early practitioners may not have fully understood the microbiological basis of periodontal disease, traditional medicine prescribed a variety of herbal products to maintain gum health and alleviate oral ailments. For instance, cool tea leaves were commonly used to reduce gingival inflammation, which was believed to be associated with excessive "stomach heat." Several herbs, including lotus leaves, tea polyphenols, Radix Zanthoxyli, and Flos Lonicerae, were widely used for their therapeutic effects.

Scientific studies have since validated some of these traditional remedies. Lotus leaf extracts, for example, have demonstrated strong antibacterial activity against common periodontal pathogens such as Aggregatibacter actinomycetemcomitans, Porphyromonas gingivalis, and Fusobacterium nucleatum. Additionally, tea polyphenols like catechins have been shown to inhibit virulence factors of Prevotella intermedia and P. gingivalis. A specific catechin called epigallocatechin has also been found to suppress matrix metalloproteinase (MMP) activity, reducing osteoclast formation and bone resorption associated with periodontal disease. Furthermore, green tea extract has been successfully incorporated into local drug delivery systems for periodontal therapy, demonstrating significant improvements in clinical parameters. A direct relationship between green tea consumption and improved periodontal health has also been proposed, suggesting that diet plays a crucial role in oral well-being.

Chewing Sticks: A Natural Toothbrush Alternative

Before the invention of modern toothbrushes, people across India and other parts of the world used chewing sticksderived from medicinal plants for oral hygiene. Some of the most commonly used chewing sticks in India are obtained from:

- Neem (Azadirachta indica)
- Mango (Mangifera indica)
- Babul (Acacia arabica)
- Guava (Psidium guajava)
- Miswak (Salvadora persica)

Miswak remains widely popular among Muslim communities in India and the Middle East. Research suggests that chewing sticks may be as effective as toothbrushes in removing dental plaque, although conclusive evidence is still lacking.

The effectiveness of chewing sticks is attributed to several factors:

- Increased Salivation – The mechanical action of chewing stimulates saliva production, which helps flush out oral bacteria and debris.
- Antibacterial Properties – Miswak has demonstrated antibacterial activity against early plaque colonizers such as streptococci and periodontal pathogens like P. gingivalis. This effect is believed to be due to tannins and thiocyanate, which are released during chewing and activate the salivary hydrogen peroxide/peroxidase/thiocyanate system, exerting a potent antimicrobial effect.
- Natural Chemical Composition – Various chewing sticks contain plant-derived antibacterial compounds. For example:
    - Neem contains isoprenoids (nimbin, nimbinin, nimbidin), chloride, and fluoride, which inhibit oral streptococci.
    - Mango contains tannins, bitter gums, and resins, known for their antimicrobial properties.
    - Many chewing sticks exhibit antioxidant activity, comparable to vitamins C and K. Neem, in particular, contains compounds such as gallic acid, gallocatechin, epigallocatechin, and catechin, which reduce oxidative stress and inflammation.

Given these benefits, chewing sticks continue to be used in many rural and traditional communities as an effective alternative to modern toothbrushes.

Tongue Cleaning: A Forgotten Yet Essential Practice

Both Indian and Chinese traditional medicine have long emphasized tongue examination as a diagnostic tool for assessing overall health. In fact, an entire chapter in the Charaka Samhita is dedicated to tongue health. Tongue cleaning has been a crucial component of oral hygiene in India, with various tools, including coconut leaves and modern stainless steel or plastic tongue cleaners, being used to remove debris and bacteria from the tongue's surface.

Scientific evidence now supports the importance of tongue cleaning in preventing periodontal disease and halitosis (bad breath). Periodontal pathogens such as A. actinomycetemcomitans have been found to colonize not just the gingival crevice but also other areas of the oral cavity, including the tongue. Tongue cleaning plays a role in full-mouth disinfection, which has been shown to be an effective strategy for plaque control and maintaining periodontal health. This traditional practice, therefore, has strong scientific backing and continues to be widely recommended by dental professionals.

Traditional Mouthwashes and Rinsing Practices

Mouthwashes have been referenced in both Indian and Chinese traditional medicine, but they were historically used more as therapeutic agents rather than as daily plaque control measures. Ayurveda describes two types of traditional mouth rinses:

1. Kavalagra – A herbal preparation made into a paste or bolus, which was then diluted into a liquid form. The individual would hold this preparation in the mouth until nasal discharge or lacrimation occurred, indicating detoxification.
2. Gandoosha – A liquid-based mouthwash, usually containing essential oils or herbal extracts. The mouth was filled three-quarters full with the rinse, which was then vigorously swished around.

Common herbal ingredients in these traditional mouth rinses included:

- Triphala (a blend of three medicinal fruits)
- Dasamoola (a combination of ten medicinal roots)
- Guggulu (Commiphora wightii, known for its anti-inflammatory properties)
- Pippali (long pepper, used for its antimicrobial effects)
- Sarshapashunti (mustard and dry ginger)

Essential oil-based mouthwashes, such as sahacharadi taila and irimedadi taila, were also used for periodontal treatment. Additionally, oil pulling with sesame oil has remained a prevalent practice in rural India. Scientific studies suggest that sesame oil has antibacterial, anti-inflammatory, and antioxidant properties. The key bioactive components in sesame oil—sesamin, sesamolin, and sesaminol—have been shown to potentiate the action of vitamin E and reduce oxidative stress. Furthermore, the polyunsaturated fatty acids in sesame oil may inhibit lipid peroxidation and help combat inflammation, making oil pulling a potentially beneficial practice for oral health.

Cultural Influence on Oral Hygiene Rituals

In Indian culture, oral hygiene is deeply intertwined with daily rituals and socio-cultural habits. Unlike Western cultures where cutlery is used, Indians traditionally eat with their hands. After meals, it is customary to rinse the mouth thoroughly—a practice observed by approximately 50% of the population, particularly among the elderly and those less influenced by Western customs.

This post-meal rinsing habit, even when performed with plain water, likely plays a crucial role in preventing food accumulation and reducing bacterial load in the mouth. In some instances, finger brushing accompanies rinsing, further aiding mechanical plaque removal. While modern mouthwashes are not a significant part of traditional Indian oral hygiene, these natural rinsing habits have likely contributed to oral cleanliness and disease prevention over centuries.

Traditional Indian oral hygiene methods, including the use of herbal remedies, chewing sticks, tongue cleaning, and oil pulling, have been practiced for millennia. Many of these methods have been scientifically validated for their antimicrobial, anti-inflammatory, and antioxidant properties. Integrating these time-honored practices with modern dentistry can help create a more holistic approach to oral health, bridging the gap between ancient wisdom and contemporary science.

Binomial	Local/English name	Family	Parts used	Traditional uses/(informants)
Acorus calamus Linn. (菖蒲 Chāng Pú)	Vacha/sweet flag	Araceae	Rhizome	Paste of the rhizome is applied to painful teeth and gums
Allium sativum Linn. (大蒜 Dà Suàn)	Lahsun/garlic	Alliaceae	Bulb	The paste of the bulb is applied to the gums and cavities of infected teeth
Bombax ceiba Linn. (木棉 Mù Mián)	Semal/silk cotton tree	Bombacaceae	Gum	Gum is used to treat toothache
Cinnamomum tamala (柴桂 Chái Guì) Nees and Eberm.	Tejpat/Indian bay leaf	Lauraceae	Stem bark	Stem bark juice is applied to the teeth to treat tooth decay and toothache
Citrus medica Linn. (佛手柑 Fó Shǒu Gān)	Nimbu/lemon	Rutaceae	Fruit	Used to treat bleeding gums in scurvy due to its high content of vitamin C
Datura stramonium Linn. (曼陀羅 Màn Tuó Luó)	Dhatura/mad apple	Solanaceae	Seeds	Seeds mixed with butter are burnt and the smoke is inhaled into the mouth
Juglans regia Linn. (胡桃 Hú Táo)	Akhoda/walnut	Juglandaceae	Oil and fruits	Oil and fruits are used in making traditional tooth powder to cure toothache and pyorrhea
Justicia adhatoda Linn.	Vasing/Malabar nut	Acanthaceae	Twigs	The twigs of the plant are used as tooth picks/brushes to treat pyorrhea
Myrica esculenta Buch.-Ham.	Kaphal/box myrtle	Myricaceae	Bark	The bark is chewed to relieve toothache
Ocimum sanctum Linn. (羅勒 Luó Lè)	Tulsi/holy basil	Lamiaceae	Leaves	Powder of dry leaves along with salt is applied to painful teeth
Phyllanthus emblica Linn. (油柑 Yóu Gān)	Amla/emblic myrobalan	Euphorbiaceae	Fruit	The fruit is a good source of vitamin C and is used to treat bleeding gums
Punica granatum Linn. (石榴 Shí Liú)	Anar/pomegranate	Punicaceae	Fruit	It is very useful in bleeding gums due to scurvy
Ricinus communis Linn. (蓖麻 Bì Má)	Arand/castorbean	Euphorbiaceae	Twigs and leaves	Tender shoots are used as toothbrushes in dental caries. Leaf juice is used to gargle in Pyorrhea
Urtica dioica Linn. (蕁麻 Qián Má)	Kandali/stinging nettle	Urticaceae	Root	Two to three drops of root extract are applied to hollow tooth cavities to treat toothache
Vitex negundo Linn. (黃荊 Huáng Jīng)	Sivali/five-leaved chaste tree	Verbenaceae	Leaves	Leaf decoction is used as a mouthwash to relieve toothache
Zanthoxylum armatum DC (秦椒 Qín Jiāo)	Timbru/bamboo-leaved prinklish ash	Rutaceae	Fruit and twig	Powder of the fruits is used as a remedy for toothache. Small twigs of the branches are used to treat toothache
Zingiber officinale Linn. (薑 Jiāng)	Adrak/ginger	Zingiberaceae	Rhizome	Paste of rhizomes is applied to the teeth to treat toothache and tooth decay

DC: De Candolle

Medicinal plants and their traditional uses for the treatment of a variety of dental problems

Biological effects of traditional Indian medicines

Herbal product	Active ingredients	Mechanism of action	Reference
Neem	Nimbin, nimbinin, nimbidin	Antibacterial effect against oral streptococci	[48,37]
	Catechins	Reduced bacterial adhesion to tooth surface	[49]
		Reduced oxidative burst from polymorphonuclear leukocytes	[38]
Guava	Essential oils, pinene, avicularin, and other polyphenols	Anti-inflammatory and antibacterial effect	[50,51]
Triphala	Amalaki, haritaki, and bibhitaki Gallic acid	Antioxidant effect Reduction in matrix metalloproteinase 9 levels	[52]
Sesame oil	Sesamin, sesamolin, and sesaminol	Antioxidant property Potentiates the action of vitamin E	[53]
Miswak	Tannins, thiocyanate	Increased salivation	
		Inhibits *Po. gingivalis*	[33]
		Activates the salivary H_2O_2/peroxidase/thiocyanate system	[34]

Dental practice in ancient Egypt

In the heart of ancient Egypt, dentistry was a blend of medical expertise, practical innovation, and spiritual belief. Healers treated toothaches with honey and herbs, priests invoked divine protection against pain, and skilled practitioners used gold wires to stabilize loose teeth. Long before modern dentistry, Egyptian physicians—known as *swnw*—developed sophisticated treatments for oral ailments, as documented in texts like the *Ebers Papyrus* and *Edwin Smith Papyrus*. Mummies reveal evidence of severe dental wear, abscesses, and decay, often caused by a coarse diet and grit from stone-ground grains. Despite these challenges, ancient Egyptian dentists pioneered techniques such as resin-based fillings and early forms of surgical intervention. Their approach to oral health, rooted in both science and spirituality, laid the foundation for some of the earliest recorded dental practices in history.

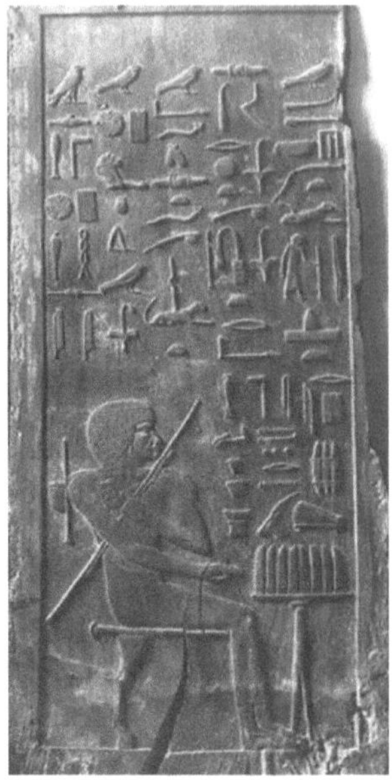

Translations of hieroglyphic inscriptions discovered in Egyptian tombs and monuments have provided insights into the occupations of the deceased, revealing instances where individuals held medical or dental titles. Among approximately 150 individuals identified as medical practitioners in ancient Egypt, only nine have been recognized specifically as dentists. These professionals appear to have been classified into two primary ranks: one described as being "concerned with teeth," likely referring to a dentist, and another titled "one who deals with teeth." The exact distinction between these titles remains uncertain, though it may indicate differences in responsibilities or professional standing. Additionally, higher-ranking dental positions such as "chief of dentists" were documented, with the most prestigious title possibly being "chief dentist of the palace."

The earliest known dentist—both in Egypt and globally—was Hesyre, whose legacy is preserved through six intricately carved wooden panels found in his tomb at Saqqara, near modern-day Cairo. These panels are regarded as some of the finest wooden artifacts from antiquity. Hesyre, who lived around 2660 BCE, was not only designated as the "chief of dentists" but also held the title of "chief of physicians," along with various other religious and administrative roles. Similarly, other dentists of the time, such as Nyanksekhmet and Khuwy, carried multiple designations. Nyanksekhmet was also referred to as a "chief of physicians," while Khuwy was identified as both a dentist and an "elder of the physicians of the palace," in addition to specializing in gastrointestinal ailments. It remains unclear whether these multiple titles indicated expertise in various fields or if they were primarily honorary or administrative in nature. Nonetheless, their existence highlights a recognized need for dental care in ancient Egypt.

Hesyre

The skeletal and mummified remains from Dynastic Egypt provide the most tangible evidence regarding ancient Egyptian dental practices. Despite examinations of tens of thousands of remains spanning over 3,000 years, direct evidence of operative dental procedures is scarce. A few cases suggest possible surgical interventions for treating dental abscesses, along with three examples of what might have been prosthetic dental work and some indications of tooth extractions. While some scholars have confidently interpreted these findings as proof of an established dental profession, others have questioned these conclusions, emphasizing the need for further analysis.

The idea of surgical treatment for dental abscesses was first proposed by Hooton in 1917, based on his radiographic and visual analysis of an ancient Egyptian mandible dating back to approximately 2500 BCE. The mandible exhibited significant tooth wear, with a pulpal exposure on the lower right first molar, accompanied by an apical infection. Hooton observed two small openings in the outer cortical plate, positioned above the mental foramen and angling toward the anterior root of the affected tooth. He argued that the symmetrical appearance, upward trajectory, and penetration depth of these holes indicated deliberate drilling, potentially to drain the abscess.

This theory was later supported by Egyptologist James Breasted, who speculated that the holes might have been created using a bronze bow drill. The bow drill was a known tool in ancient Egypt, primarily employed for woodworking and stone carving, as depicted in 18th Dynasty tomb paintings at Luxor, particularly in the tomb of Rekhmire.

However, this interpretation faced criticism. Wingate-Todd suggested that one of the openings was merely an accessory mental foramen, while the other was a pathological cavity resulting from the abscess itself. Similarly, Leek, upon examining another ancient Egyptian mandible with comparable wear and infection, noted that its circular perforations were exceptionally well-defined and extended through intact bone tissue. The trajectory of these holes, moving from behind forward, would have required a right-angled drill—a tool that did not exist in Dynastic Egypt. He concluded that the perforations were more likely the result of bone erosion due to pus accumulation rather than surgical intervention. Furthermore, his broader analysis of skulls revealed that abscess-related bone channels formed in various orientations, undermining the argument that an upward trajectory was indicative of intentional drilling.

Additional skepticism came from Nickol et al., who argued that for such procedures to be deliberate, ancient Egyptians would have needed an advanced understanding of the pathology and anatomy of apical periodontitis—an unlikely scenario. They also suggested that Hooton's conclusions might have been influenced by early 20th-century dental practices, particularly the now-obsolete method of "apical airing," which involved similar techniques for treating abscesses.

Among the alleged dental prosthetics from ancient Egypt, the most well-known example is a mandibular second molar connected to a worn third molar by gold wire. This artifact, found in a burial shaft near Giza dating to approximately 2500 BCE, was notably discovered separately from a skull. The original dental report suggested that the teeth likely belonged to the same individual, given their similar anatomical structure and coloration. The third molar's roots showed signs of significant resorption, likely due to an inflammatory condition that caused mobility. To stabilize the tooth, it may have been secured to the adjacent second molar using gold wiring.

This finding has been widely debated, with some experts arguing that it serves as evidence of early dental prosthetics, while others suggest it may have been placed post-mortem, either for ritualistic reasons or as part of burial customs. Regardless, such discoveries provide intriguing insights into ancient Egyptian dental practices, highlighting both their medical ingenuity and the ongoing mysteries surrounding their approach to oral health care.

Leek, upon later examining the dental appliance, identified several issues with the initial conclusions. He observed that the significant wear on the teeth had altered their morphology to such an extent that accurately determining their original position in the dentition or confirming whether they belonged to the same individual was impossible. Additionally, since the third molar displayed more extensive wear compared to the second molar—despite erupting roughly six years later—it was unlikely that both teeth came from the same person. He also pointed out that the gold tubular wire, measuring only 0.35 mm in diameter, would have been too fragile to provide even temporary stability.

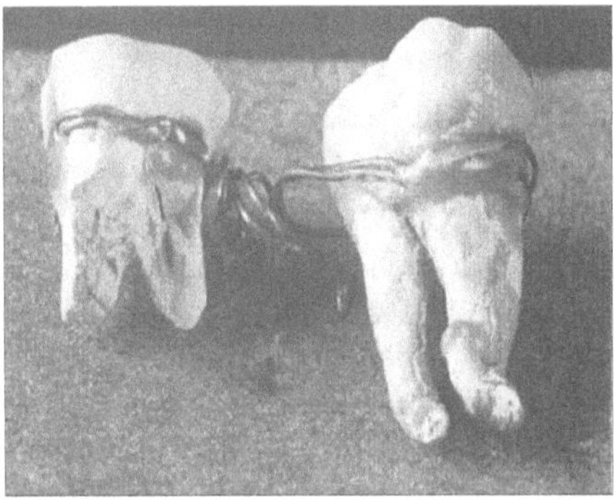

Giza bridge

Overall, the evidence suggests that this appliance was not used during the individual's lifetime. A plausible explanation is that it was inserted post-mortem, possibly to restore the body's completeness for the afterlife, a common practice in ancient Egypt. Alternatively, the teeth may have been worn as an amulet, believed to grant power or protection to the wearer.

A second dental appliance, dating to approximately 2500 BCE, was discovered at el-Quatta near Cairo. Like the previous example, it was not found in situ but was instead retrieved from the fragmented remains of a skull. This appliance consisted of a maxillary right canine encircled by a double strand of gold wire, with the ends tied in a knot on its distal surface. Separate from this were a central and lateral incisor, connected by similar gold wiring. It was initially suggested that the central incisor had been attached to the canine via a hook in the wire. The incisor featured a hole drilled in a mesiodistal direction, as well as a groove on the labial surface of the crown, designed to accommodate the gold wire. Likewise, the lateral incisor had a similar groove where the wire rested, and both teeth displayed evidence of scraping and polishing, indicating artificial modification.

This arrangement led to the theory that the canine served as an abutment for a four-unit bridge, with the central and lateral incisors acting as pontics and a missing left central incisor functioning as the other abutment. The presence of calculus on both the lateral incisor and canine was interpreted as evidence that the appliance had been worn for an extended period during life. However, several factors challenge this conclusion. The roots of the central and lateral incisors, although slightly modified, were not sufficiently adapted to function as a conventional bridge. The excessive length of the pontics would have likely caused food impaction and irritation of the surrounding mucosa. Additionally, the gold wire connecting the teeth would have been too delicate to provide adequate stability for normal chewing.

The presence of calculus on the roots might instead indicate periodontal disease during the individual's lifetime, accompanied by gingival recession and pocket formation. One possibility is that the teeth were accidentally dislodged during the mummification process and later reattached. Another scenario is that the teeth had been lost earlier in life and were replaced post-mortem, perhaps for ritualistic purposes.

The third and most significant dental appliance was found at Tura el-Asmant and is the only one discovered in situ, still attached to a skull. Dated to the Greek (Ptolemaic) period of Egyptian history (332–330 BCE), this prosthetic device featured a single pontic—a right maxillary central incisor—secured in place by a silver wire threaded through two holes drilled mesiodistally through the crown. However, the exact method of attachment to adjacent teeth remains unknown.

Radiographic analysis revealed no radiolucency above the pontic and indicated that the tooth's root was unusually short, suggesting that the tooth had been extracted, modified outside the body, and then reinserted. Further evidence of alveolar bone reshaping supported the idea that the prosthetic was placed after healing. The orientation of the drill holes implies that the procedure was performed outside the mouth rather than as an intraoral surgery.

Blustein et al. observed that the lower central incisor was positioned more labially than the adjacent teeth, which could have resulted in trauma to the upper right central incisor, possibly leading to its loss. This appliance, therefore, appears to be a genuine dental prosthesis, making it the earliest known example from ancient Egypt. However, given the extensive trade and cultural exchange during the Ptolemaic period, it remains uncertain whether this technique originated in Egypt or was introduced from elsewhere. Similar dental work has been uncovered in Sidon, Greece, and Etruscan burial sites, suggesting possible foreign influence.

The question of whether tooth extractions were performed in ancient Egypt remains unresolved. While there is substantial evidence of ante-mortem tooth loss, many of these cases appear to have resulted from periodontal disease, with teeth potentially being lost due to natural displacement or simple digital pressure. No known ancient Egyptian instruments resemble the extraction forceps found in Greek and Roman archaeological sites. However, the possibility of primitive extractions using a basic metal lever cannot be ruled out, as such tools may have been excavated but not recognized as dental instruments.

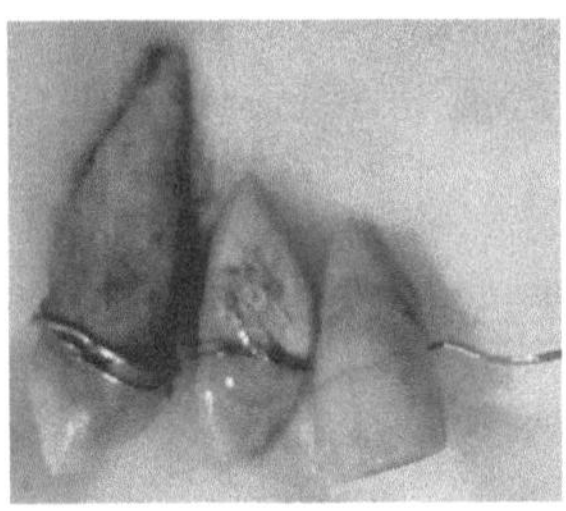

Examinations of skeletal remains have led some researchers to propose that extractions were indeed performed. Their conclusions are based on the spacing, angulation of adjacent teeth, and the contouring of alveolar bone in areas of missing dentition. However, numerous examples exist where periodontally compromised teeth were left in place, despite their likely association with pain and infection. This raises the question of why extractions, which would have provided significant pain relief, were not routinely carried out—especially given the advanced medical and surgical knowledge of the ancient Egyptians.

Section 3: Future of smile

Chapter :7: Modern smile and future of smile in changing world

The roots of cosmetic dentistry do not lie merely in clinical settings but are deeply entwined with culture, cinema, and the desire for perfection. One of the most defining moments in the birth of modern cosmetic dentistry began not in a dental clinic, but on the silver screens of early Hollywood.

The 1920s: The Era of Transformation

The 1920s marked a revolutionary shift in the entertainment industry. Silent films were giving way to "talkies," and actors—now under closer scrutiny by both cameras and audiences—had to meet new aesthetic standards. A charming smile became as essential as acting skill.

Enter Dr. Charles Pincus, a Los Angeles-based dentist with a flair for innovation. Recognizing the insecurities of actors about their dental appearance, Pincus began experimenting with ways to give them a picture-perfect smile. In 1928, he developed what would become the first set of veneers—thin porcelain covers placed on the front surface of teeth to improve appearance temporarily. These were adhered using denture glue and could only last through a few hours of filming. Yet, the impact was monumental.

Actors like Judy Garland, James Dean, and even Shirley Temple were some of the early beneficiaries of these temporary veneers. Their polished, white smiles soon became the ideal image for beauty and charisma, setting a standard that would ripple across generations.

Pincus likely didn't realize it then, but his invention planted the seed for what would grow into a billion-dollar industry. The idea that teeth could be modified not only for health but also for aesthetic purposes was groundbreaking. Over time, advancements in composite resins, ceramics, and bonding techniques allowed for permanent cosmetic treatments that were once considered impossible.

By the late 20th century, cosmetic procedures such as dental bleaching, bonding, veneers, invisible braces, and full smile makeovers became widely accessible—not only to celebrities but to everyday people seeking self-confidence through their smile.

Today, the legacy of Dr. Pincus lives on in every confident grin that flashes under a camera flash or in a mirror. Cosmetic dentistry has moved from film sets to homes, from vanity to empowerment.

What began as a quick fix for a child star has evolved into one of the most desired aspects of modern dentistry. The future of cosmetic dentistry now integrates digital smile design, 3D printing, and AI-driven diagnostics, but its heart still lies in a very human desire: to smile without hesitation.

The journey from primitive dental tools to porcelain veneers began with necessity and evolved through innovation. As chronicled in the story of Dr. Charles Pincus and the birth of cosmetic dentistry in early Hollywood, the smile transitioned from a biological function to a symbol of confidence, status, and personal identity. Today, this evolution continues, driven by digital technologies, aesthetic demands, and a deeper understanding of psychology and cultural expression.

Modern smiles are not just white and straight—they are digitally designed, customized to facial harmony, and increasingly viewed as reflections of well-being and social success (Goldstein, 2009). The integration of Digital Smile Design (DSD), CAD/CAM systems, and minimally invasive procedures has revolutionized both the precision and personalization of smile transformations (Coachman et al., 2017). Moreover, the global demand for aesthetic dentistry reflects changing societal values, where the smile is now a form of self-expression and empowerment.

As we look ahead, the future smile may incorporate AI-based diagnostics, regenerative materials, and bioengineered enamel, blurring the lines between nature and innovation. The smile—once fixed for film—now adapts to the fast-paced, image-conscious world we inhabit.

The Rise of Aesthetic Dentistry: A Cultural and Historical Perspective

In contemporary society, the pursuit of aesthetics has emerged as a central component of self-expression, especially in an era characterized by rapid globalization and evolving cultural norms. The demand for aesthetic enhancements has significantly influenced the field of dentistry, transforming it from a traditionally pain-associated discipline to one that is now closely linked with beauty, fashion, and confidence. With the rise of millennial and Gen Z populations—generations that place substantial value on physical appearance, personal branding, and social media presence—the landscape of dentistry has shifted to meet these aesthetic expectations.

Historically, dental clinics were perceived as spaces associated with discomfort, anxiety, and clinical intervention. However, modern advancements and changing societal perceptions have led to a paradigm shift. Dentistry has become increasingly associated with enhancing facial aesthetics, boosting self-esteem, and aligning with broader fashion trends. In today's social climate, individuals constantly seek novel ways to enhance their looks and distinguish themselves from others, often striving to set unique style statements. This shift in perception has made aesthetic dentistry an integral part of personal grooming and social identity.

Various cosmetic and decorative dental procedures have gained popularity over the years. These range from minimally invasive non-surgical enhancements to more elaborate surgical modifications, all aimed at improving dental aesthetics and overall facial harmony. Among the non-surgical options are decorative innovations such as tooth jewellery, dental grills, removable tooth ornaments, dental tattoos, and tooth rings. These procedures serve not only as fashion statements but also as forms of self-expression and cultural identity. When applied properly by trained professionals, such accessories can add a unique element to one's smile and boost individual confidence.

Tooth jewellery, in particular, has seen a surge in demand, especially among younger demographics. This decorative practice involves the placement of small gems or metal pieces on the surface of the teeth, usually anterior teeth, and is viewed as a symbol of boldness and uniqueness. Such procedures are considered safe when performed under sterile and professional conditions and are gaining recognition for their role in personal aesthetic enhancement.

Historically, the modification of teeth for aesthetic, cultural, or ritualistic purposes is not a new phenomenon. Evidence from ancient civilizations highlights the diverse roles dental modifications have played across time. For instance, the Mayan civilization is known for embedding jade and turquoise inlays into their anterior teeth, which was believed to offer spiritual protection and reflect high social status. In certain tribal communities, anterior teeth were intentionally extracted for functional, linguistic, or cultural purposes. For example, the removal of front teeth was believed to facilitate feeding in cases of tetanus-induced lockjaw, while in other cultures, it was associated with distinct language phonetics or as preparation for battle.

Several African tribes practiced anterior tooth extraction as part of initiation rites or for tactical reasons—such as enabling a stronger blow through a blowpipe weapon known as the *Sumpitan*. In Australia, Aboriginal communities removed teeth during rites of passage to symbolize mourning or religious transformation. In China, ancient women used a mixture of tannin and ferrous acetate to blacken their teeth, which denoted marital status and societal maturity.

Other practices across the world illustrate the multifaceted reasons behind dental modification. In Nigeria, tattooing of the lips and gingiva was customary before marriage, symbolizing maturity and social readiness. In contrast, certain South American tribes modified their teeth into sharp, pointed forms to resemble the piranha—a symbolic representation of strength and aggression. Similarly, tribes in Africa shaped their teeth to mimic fierce animals like crocodiles or tigers, thereby enhancing their visual intimidation in both warfare and social settings.

In Pre-Columbian Mesoamerican civilizations, dental filing was performed with stone tools, primarily as an act of reverence toward the solar deity, often depicted with stylized, filed teeth. Tribes from regions like Java, Sumatra, and Borneo believed that such dental alterations could ward off ancestral spirits and help secure safe passage into the afterlife. In these cultures, tooth filing was seen as a harmonizing act between physical beauty and spiritual fulfillment.

In addition to non-surgical modifications, various surgical aesthetic procedures have also emerged within modern dental and maxillofacial practices. These include procedures such as oral piercings (tongue, lip, and cheek piercings), lip reduction, lip repositioning, and lip augmentation. These surgical interventions are typically pursued for either aesthetic refinement or functional correction and are becoming increasingly common among individuals seeking customized alterations to their orofacial appearance.

Together, these practices—both ancient and modern—reflect the profound intersection of dentistry with art, culture, identity, and self-expression. The aesthetic aspect of dentistry today transcends its traditional medical purpose, embracing a more holistic role that encompasses beauty, cultural symbolism, and psychological well-being. As trends continue to evolve, so too will the scope and techniques of aesthetic dentistry, marking an ongoing transformation in how we perceive and interact with our smiles.

Non-Surgical Aesthetic Dental Modifications

The domain of non-surgical aesthetic dentistry has witnessed remarkable growth, offering individuals numerous ways to enhance their smiles without undergoing invasive procedures. Building upon ancient and contemporary practices, these modifications reflect a blend of cultural expression, personal identity, and modern fashion trends. Among these innovations are tooth jewellery, tooth gems, tooth studs, tooth rings, tooth tattoos, and dental grills—each serving as a medium of self-expression while adding a unique visual element to the dentition.

One of the earliest references to decorative dental modifications can be found in Indian mythology. The Mahabharata, an ancient Indian epic, recounts an incident from the Battle of Kurukshetra where Lord Krishna, disguised as a Brahmin, requests gold from Karna. In a display of selflessness, Karna offers his gold-filled teeth, suggesting that dental ornamentation was practiced as early as 2500 BCE, not only for aesthetics but also as a symbol of virtue and sacrifice.

Tooth Gems and Tooth Jewellery

Tooth gems are modern decorative accessories made from glass crystals set on thin aluminum foil, available in a variety of shapes, sizes, and colors. These include round crystals, alphabet designs, and jewel tones such as ruby, sapphire, aquamarine, emerald green, and pink. Popular brands like *Skyce* and *Sapphire crystals* (Ivoclar Vivadent AG, Schaan, Liechtenstein) are known for their high-quality materials. Skyce, being transparent, adds a subtle glint to the smile, while Sapphire offers white and blue tones.

The procedure for applying these gems is non-invasive, painless, and reversible, typically requiring only 10–15 minutes. Since it does not involve drilling or tooth preparation, the gem can be removed or replaced at any time without damaging the enamel. These gems can also be strategically placed on areas of enamel hypoplasia or pigmentation, serving both cosmetic and corrective purposes. Common diameters include 1.8 mm and 2.6 mm, with rainbow crystals being the most economical and suitable for short-term use.

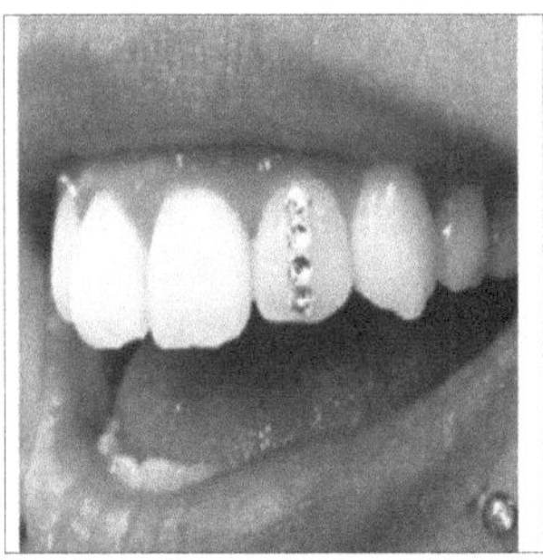

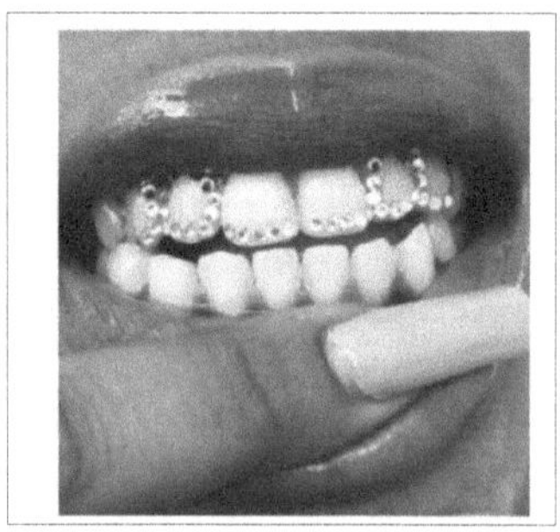

Tooth stud

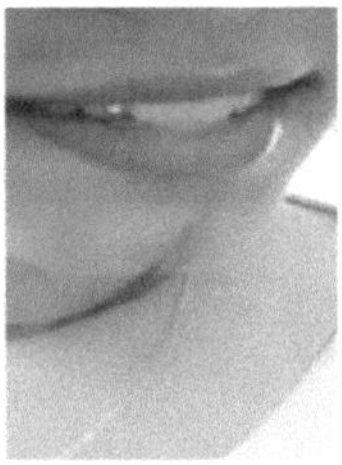

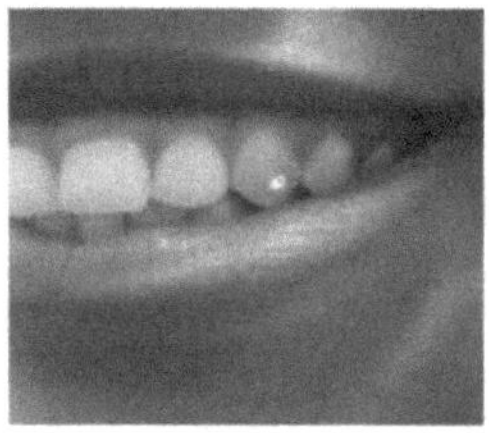

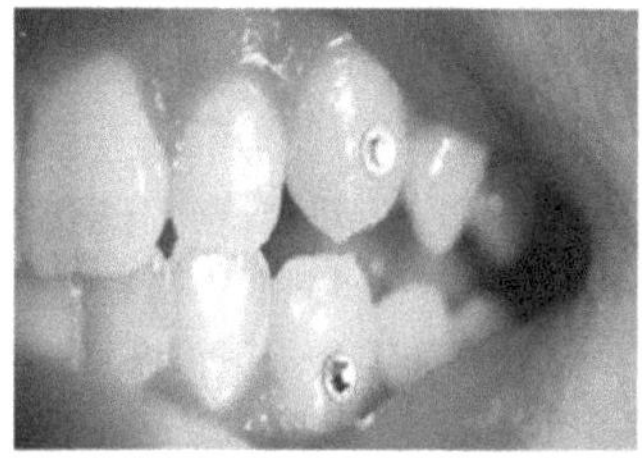

Tooth studs, also known as Twinkles, are another form of dental ornamentation composed of 24-carat gold or white gold, often embedded with precious stones like diamonds, sapphires, or rubies. These studs feature an attachment mechanism similar to orthodontic brackets, allowing them to adhere securely to the enamel. They are most commonly affixed to the maxillary incisors or canines, and like tooth gems, they are painless to apply and typically completed within 15 minutes.

Tooth Rings

Tooth rings involve the creation of a small, polished hole on the disto-incisal edge of a maxillary central incisor. Through this hole, a decorative ring—often embedded with gemstones—is suspended. The selection of ring diameter must consider the patient's overjet and occlusion to avoid any interference with bite function. In some custom designs, rings may connect adjacent teeth (e.g., between central and lateral incisors), enhancing the uniqueness of the accessory.

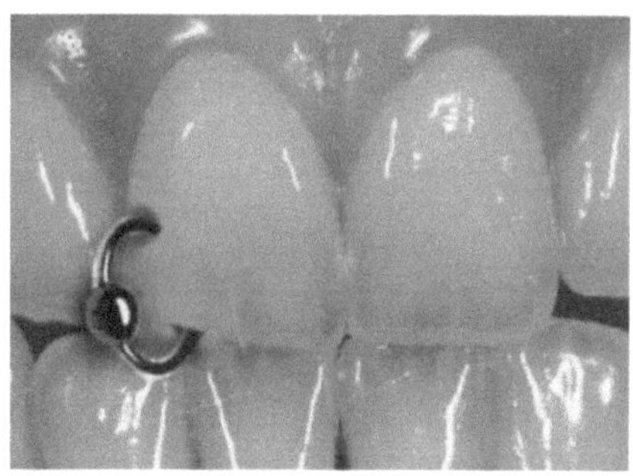

Tooth Tattoos

Although the term "tooth tattoo" is a misnomer (as traditional tattoos involve dermal pigmentation), dental tattoos refer to customized graphics or illustrations applied to the lab-fabricated dental crown prior to cementation. These designs range from symbols of religion, celebrities, and floral motifs to animals and loyalty emblems, tailored to personal tastes and cultural affiliations. The age group most inclined towards this trend typically falls between 14–35 years.

Tooth tattoos can be temporary or permanent. Temporary tattoos are applied using stencil-based techniques that adhere to the crown surface, while permanent versions require enamel reduction for crown placement. The procedure takes around 15–20 minutes and was popularized in mainstream culture by hip-hop artists and celebrities in the early 2000s.

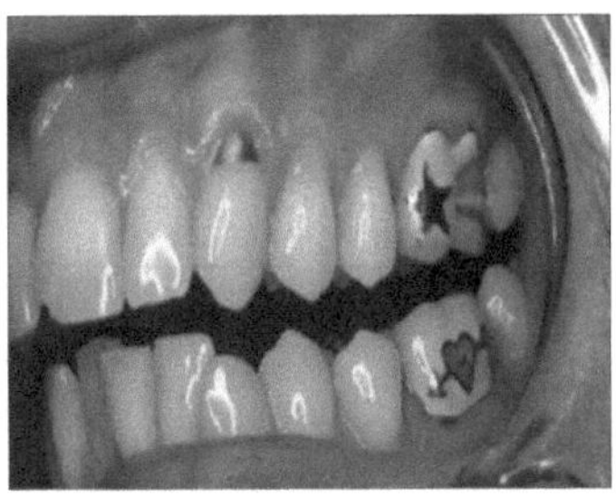

Dental Grills

Dental grills, or "grillz", represent one of the most extravagant forms of dental ornamentation. These are often crafted from precious metals like gold or platinum and may be encrusted with diamonds or other gemstones. Unlike other aesthetic procedures that focus on subtlety, grills are designed to cover the entire visible anterior dentition, offering a bold, flamboyant look. Popularized by American rap and hip-hop culture, grills are worn as fashion statements, reflecting status, wealth, and individual style.

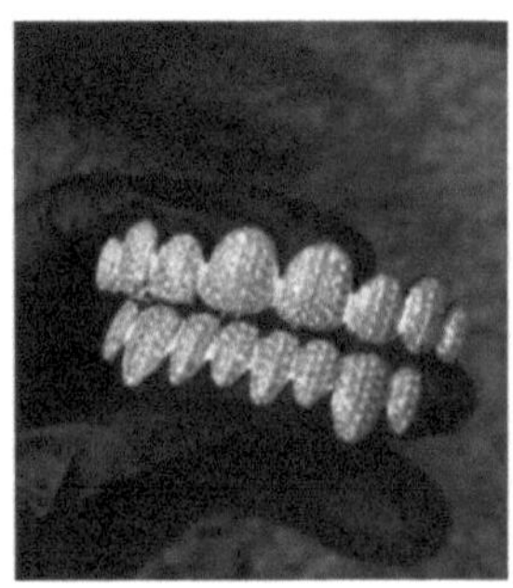

Surgical Aesthetic Modifications in Dentistry

While non-surgical enhancements continue to dominate aesthetic dentistry, surgical interventions have carved a niche of their own, particularly in the domain of oral and facial piercings. These procedures, although invasive, are becoming increasingly popular among individuals seeking distinctive and personalized forms of self-expression. The oral cavity, due to its visibility and symbolic association with communication and identity, is a frequent site for such modifications.

Oral Piercing

Oral piercing involves the perforation of soft tissues in and around the mouth to place decorative jewellery. It is a more invasive form of aesthetic alteration compared to enamel-based embellishments and requires strict aseptic techniques and post-operative care. Depending on the anatomical site, various types of piercings and associated terminologies are used:

- Tongue Piercing: Placement through the midline of the tongue, typically in the anterior third.
- Monroe Piercing: On the upper lip (left side), named after Marilyn Monroe.
- Madonna Piercing: On the upper lip (right side), referencing the pop icon.
- Labret Piercing: On the lower lip, often central.
- Medusa Piercing: In the philtrum, the vertical groove in the upper lip.
- Dimple Piercing: On the cheeks, mimicking natural dimples.
- Smiley Piercing: Through the maxillary labial frenum.
- Frowny Piercing: On the mandibular labial frenum.
- Web Piercing: On the lingual frenum beneath the tongue.
- Rhino Piercing: Typically refers to nasal piercings with vertical alignment.
- Uvula Piercing: Performed on the uvula, though rare and highly risky.

The commonly used jewellery includes studs, barbells, and rings, and must be crafted from biocompatible materialssuch as surgical-grade stainless steel, niobium, titanium, or surgical gold to reduce allergic reactions and enhance healing.

Tongue Piercing

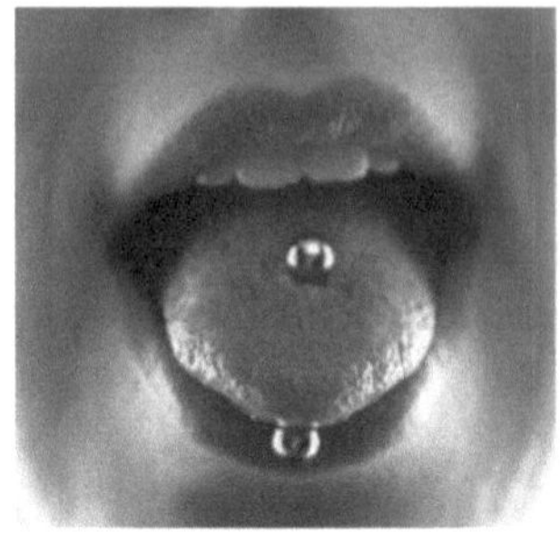

Historically, tongue piercing holds deep ritualistic and spiritual significance. Among the Mayan civilization (circa 700 BCE) and later the Aztecs, tongue piercing was considered a sacred ritual reserved for priests and royalty, symbolizing sacrifice and communication with deities. This practice largely diminished following Spanish colonization in 1521 [17].

In modern contexts, tongue piercing involves vertically inserting a barbell-shaped ornament through the tongue, typically at the midline of the anterior third. A larger temporary barbell is used initially to accommodate post-piercing edema. The procedure is performed under aseptic conditions using a sterile piercing needle. The jewellery is placed from the ventral to dorsal surface, and the visible end is secured by screwing a ball onto the post. Healing typically occurs within 4 to 6 weeks, provided there are no complications such as infection, excessive swelling, or trauma to adjacent teeth.

Tongue Splitting

Another extreme and controversial body modification is tongue splitting (also known as "tongue bifurcation"), in which the tongue is surgically divided to create a bifid or forked appearance, mimicking the tongue of reptiles. Some individuals view this as a form of avant-garde body art and personal transformation.

While surgical tongue splitting can be performed by trained professionals using scalpel-based incisions followed by suturing, there are instances where individuals attempt non-medical self-splitting techniques, such as:

- Using a blade or cautery pen without anesthesia.
- Tying a fishing line through a punctured tongue and gradually tightening it to sever the tissue.

To prevent the split edges from healing back together, the individual may manually stretch the tongue segments apartduring the healing period. Improper techniques can result in excessive bleeding, infection, nerve damage, speech impairment, and long-term scarring. Often, secondary corrective surgeries are necessary to reshape or address healing complications

The Role of Dental Veneers in Modern Cosmetic Dentistry

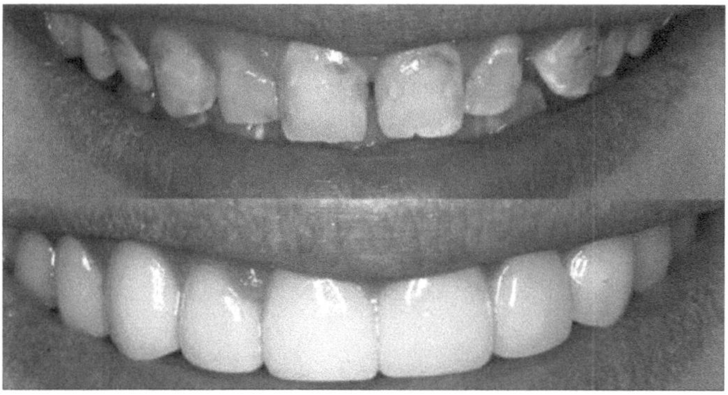

Dental veneers are thin, custom-crafted shells designed to cover the front surface of teeth. Typically made from porcelain or composite resin, these materials are designed to replicate the light-reflecting qualities of natural teeth. Veneers are commonly used to enhance the appearance of teeth that are discolored, worn, chipped, slightly misaligned, or have noticeable gaps.

Types of Veneers

Dental veneers generally fall into two categories:

- **Porcelain Veneers:** Renowned for their durability and natural look, porcelain veneers resist stains and offer long-lasting results. They are fabricated in dental labs and require more tooth preparation compared to their composite counterparts.
- **Composite Veneers:** Made from tooth-colored resin, composite veneers are applied directly to the teeth and sculpted in place. While not as strong as porcelain, they are more budget-friendly and can often be completed in a single visit.

Applications of Dental Veneers

Dental veneers are highly versatile and can address a wide range of aesthetic concerns:

- **Discoloration:** For teeth that don't respond to whitening, veneers offer a bright and consistent shade.
- **Worn Teeth:** Age-related wear and damage, such as erosion or chipping, can be covered with veneers for a refreshed look.
- **Chips and Cracks:** Minor surface damage is easily concealed, restoring a smooth, natural appearance.
- **Misalignment and Gaps:** Veneers can visually correct minor misalignment or spacing issues, offering a straighter smile without orthodontics.
- **Irregular Shape or Size:** Uneven or disproportionate teeth can be reshaped to achieve balance and symmetry.

Benefits of Dental Veneers

Veneers are a popular choice in cosmetic dentistry thanks to their numerous advantages:

- **Enhanced Aesthetics:** Veneers closely resemble natural teeth in translucency and color, creating a radiant and attractive smile.
- **Stain Resistance:** Especially in the case of porcelain veneers, resistance to staining from food, drinks, and smoking helps maintain a bright appearance.

Common Myths About Veneers

Despite their benefits, several myths about veneers persist:

- **Myth 1: Veneers Look Artificial**
  Thanks to modern dental advancements, veneers now look incredibly natural. Experienced dentists ensure veneers blend seamlessly with your existing teeth in color, shape, and translucency.
- **Myth 2: Veneers Are Only for Celebrities**
  While veneers were once seen as a luxury reserved for public figures, the have become much more accessible and affordable for the general public.

- **Myth 3: The Procedure Is Painful**
  Veneer application is typically pain-free, involving minimal tooth preparation and often performed under local anesthesia. Most patients experience little to no discomfort.

- **Myth 4: Extensive Tooth Shaving Is Necessary**
  Modern techniques are minimally invasive, often requiring only slight enamel removal for proper fit and a natural look.

Cultural Shift Towards the "Perfect Smile": A Scientific Perspective

Over the past few decades, there has been a significant cultural transformation in the perception of an ideal smile, shifting from a mere functional aspect of oral health to a symbol of beauty, confidence, and social status. This evolution is deeply rooted in psychological, societal, and media-driven influences that have reshaped public expectations and clinical approaches in dentistry.

Historically, the function of teeth and oral structures was primarily valued for mastication, phonation, and general health. However, with the advancement of aesthetic dentistry and increased awareness about facial aesthetics, the smile has become an important non-verbal communication tool, influencing first impressions, social interactions, and self-esteem .

Modern media, including television, cinema, and social platforms, has played a critical role in idealizing white, symmetrical, and aligned teeth as the norm. The portrayal of celebrities and influencers with "perfect" smiles has contributed to the increasing demand for cosmetic dental procedures, such as veneers, teeth whitening, orthodontics, and smile design [3,4]. A study by Mehl et al. demonstrated that symmetrical tooth alignment and whiteness significantly enhance perceived attractiveness, reinforcing the preference for the standardized "Hollywood smile" .

In addition, the psychosocial impact of dental appearance is now well-documented. Numerous studies have found that individuals with esthetically pleasing smiles are perceived as more intelligent, successful, and socially competent [6]. According to Newton et al., dissatisfaction with dental appearance is positively associated with low self-esteem and increased anxiety in social settings, further driving the desire for aesthetic dental interventions.

Culturally, this shift is not confined to Western societies. There is a growing trend across Asian and African countries to conform to global aesthetic standards. For example, in countries like South Korea, Japan, and India, the market for cosmetic dental procedures has expanded significantly due to the rising influence of beauty standards and increasing dental awareness .

Moreover, the economic implications of this trend are notable. The global cosmetic dentistry market is projected to reach USD 30 billion by 2026, underscoring how societal values have transformed oral health from necessity to luxury and self-expression .

This cultural shift has also posed ethical considerations for dental professionals, who must now balance clinical necessity with patient-driven aesthetic demands. Understanding the cultural psychology behind this phenomenon enables clinicians to approach aesthetic treatments with sensitivity and patient-centered care.

Impact of technology

Digital smile designing

A smile is a refined neuromuscular activity that involves the coordinated contraction and relaxation of several facial muscles. Key muscles include the zygomaticus major and minor, levator labii superioris, depressor anguli oris, and the risorius. These work synergistically with the orbicularis oris, which encircles the mouth and forms the core musculature at the lip commissures. All of these muscles are innervated by the facial nerve (cranial nerve VII), facilitating both involuntary and voluntary expressions [6].

Human smiles are typically categorized into two distinct types:

1. Genuine (Duchenne) Smile – This occurs spontaneously and reflects true emotion. It involves strong activation of both the zygomatic major (raising the corners of the mouth) and orbicularis oculi (creating crow's feet near the eyes).

2. Social (Non-Duchenne) Smile – This is a conscious, polite gesture, primarily engaging the zygomatic major, and is often used in social settings to convey friendliness or acknowledgment.

The visible zone during smiling—termed the smile or display zone—was described by Ackermann et al. [7]. It is demarcated by the upper and lower lips and frames the exposure of teeth and gingiva. Key elements influencing this zone include:

- Lip thickness
- Width between lip commissures
- Interlabial distance
- Smile index (ratio of width to height)
- Gingival curvature and health

The "smile arc", created by the curvature of the maxillary anterior incisal edges, ideally follows the contour of the lower lip, enhancing esthetic appeal.

Fundamentals of Smile Designing

Creating an ideal smile involves a comprehensive understanding of facial musculature, proportions, and esthetic parameters. Although digital smile design (DSD) software can assist in planning, clinical success depends on a multidisciplinary approach—involving orthodontics, prosthodontics, periodontics, and, in some cases, orthognathic and plastic surgery [9].

Critical facial considerations in smile design include:

- Facial symmetry: Optimal esthetics demand bilateral harmony.
- Facial profile: The anteroposterior alignment of facial bones affects smile visibility.
- Facial vertical thirds: The face should ideally divide into three equal vertical segments:
    - From glabella to superciliary arch
    - From arch to nasal tip
    - From subnasale to menton

The intercanthal (interpupillary) line should be perpendicular to the Frankfurt horizontal plane, ensuring proper orientation of facial elements.

From a dental perspective, approximately 2 mm of the maxillary central incisors should be visible during a normal smile, with interdental papillae subtly exposed [11]. Excessive gingival display leads to a "gummy smile," while insufficient exposure flattens the philtrum and may mimic a frown.

Dental Composition and Esthetic Ratios

The maxillary central incisors significantly influence smile harmony. Research indicates the ideal width-to-length ratiolies between 0.75 and 0.80, with slight dominance of the central incisors preferred over adjacent teeth .

To achieve proportional harmony, several mathematical and esthetic theories have been introduced:

- Golden Proportion (Lombardi) – Suggests the apparent width of each anterior tooth decreases in a specific ratio from the central incisor to the canine.
- Recurring Esthetic Dental Proportion (Ward) – Emphasizes repeated ratios in anterior tooth widths.
- M Proportions (Méthot) and Chu's Esthetic Gauges – Offer quantifiable guidelines for tooth dimensions and relationships.

Additional esthetic landmarks that influence smile design include:

- Dental midline alignment
- Crown height and width
- Zenith points (most apical part of the gingival margin)
- Axial inclinations
- Interdental papilla height
- Contact area proportions

Evolution of Smile Designing Technologies

The journey from manual sketches to high-end digital simulation has transformed smile designing dramatically:

- Generation 1: Initial designs were drawn manually using markers on patient photographs, offering basic visual references but lacking correlation with intraoral models.
- Generation 2: With digital tools like Microsoft Paint or PowerPoint, more accurate tracings could be overlaid on photographs and compared with models.
- Generation 3: Two-dimensional (2D) digital designs began integrating with wax-ups—physical mock-ups of the planned smile.
- Generation 4: Development of algorithm-based 3D facial analysis allowed a more comprehensive understanding of esthetic parameters and facial dynamics.
- Generation 5: Introduction of intraoral scanners replaced conventional impressions, improving precision in digital modeling.
- Generation 6: The latest advancement includes 4D smile design using technologies like MODJAW, which captures jaw movement in real time and merges it with CAD/CAM systems. This allows clinicians to predict esthetic outcomes dynamically, reducing the need for invasive procedures and revisions .

Digital Smile Design: Evolution and Application

The advent of digitalization has significantly influenced various professional fields, including dentistry. Digital Smile Design (DSD), introduced by Brazilian dentist Christian Coachman in 2007, represents a revolutionary tool in esthetic dentistry. It allows clinicians to digitally design a patient's smile using a comprehensive set of pre- and post-treatment photographs. This technique not only enhances treatment accuracy but also improves patient communication and satisfaction by actively involving them in the decision-making process [18].

DSD provides an interactive platform that enables clinicians to present potential treatment outcomes to patients, gather their preferences, and collaboratively determine the best course of action. Coachman and Calamita described DSD as a versatile, multipurpose analytical software, capable of conducting a meticulous analysis of both facial and dental features that may otherwise be missed by conventional examination or static photography [19].

Requirements for Digital Smile Design

Several tools and technologies are integral to the DSD process:

- Software platforms: Adobe Photoshop, Microsoft PowerPoint, Smile Designer Pro (Tasty Tech Ltd.), Aesthetic Digital Smile Design (ADSD by Dr. Valerio Bini), DSD App (Coachman), Apple Keynote, NemoDSD (3D), Exocad DentalCAD.
- Hardware and tools: A digital SLR camera, intraoral scanner for digital impressions, CAD/CAM processing machines for 3D printing.

The process begins with capturing digital impressions of both arches using intraoral scanners. These are uploaded to CAD/CAM software for rendering and 3D printing. Additionally, high-resolution facial photographs—including profile and frontal views—and videos capturing the dynamic interplay of teeth, gingiva, lips, and facial musculature are essential. These records serve as the blueprint for smile design.

The three fundamental photographic views used in DSD include:

1. Full facial view with a natural smile.
2. Resting facial posture.
3. Intraoral view of maxillary and mandibular arches without occlusion.

A 1:1 magnified image of the central incisor on a black background provides detailed reference data for the dental technician. Videos can be integrated into presentations to help visualize the patient's dynamic expressions.

Commercially available DSD software includes: CEREC Smile Design (Sirona), Digital Smile System (DSS), Smile Design Pro (Tasty Tech), G Design (Hack Dental), Romexis Smile Design (Planmeca), and Smile Composer (3Shape) .

DSD Workflow: Step-by-Step

The Digital Smile Design process follows a systematic protocol to ensure precision and esthetic harmony:

1. Initial Scan & Import: The patient's dentition is digitally scanned using an intraoral scanner and imported into the chosen DSD software.
2. Facial Photograph Calibration:
    - Facial images are uploaded, and two perpendicular lines (horizontal and vertical) are drawn at the center, creating a digital reference point (a "+" sign) at the level of the anterior teeth with lips apart.
    - The interpupillary line is used to establish horizontal reference, acting as a digital facebow.
3. Soft Tissue Evaluation:
    - Gingival contours, lip dynamics, and facial lines are grouped and digitally superimposed over the facial image for thorough analysis.
4. Tooth Template Placement:
    - A standard tooth template is overlaid on the image to assess axial inclination, proportions, and alignmentwith neighboring teeth and soft tissue outlines.
5. Intraoral Verification:
    - A retracted intraoral view is examined to ensure the intraoral image aligns with facial reference baselines using three horizontal lines:
        - Line 1: Intercanine width (from cusp tip to cusp tip).
        - Line 2: Middle third of central incisor to adjacent incisal edge.
        - Line 3: From philtrum to interdental papilla and incisal embrasure.

6. Proportion Analysis:
    - Using rectangular cropping tools, the width-to-length ratio of central incisors is analyzed for symmetry and balance.
7. Digital Morphing & Editing:
    - The tooth template is digitally adapted using morphing tools to align with esthetic objectives. Patient preferences can be incorporated at this stage for a personalized design.
8. Calibrating Real Dimensions:
    - A digital ruler tool is used to record actual measurements from the 3D model and sync them within the software, ensuring precision in gingival contour, incisal edges, and attached gingiva.
9. Transferring the Design to the Cast:
    - Using calipers, baseline points are transferred from the image to the cast. Horizontal lines indicating the gingival margins and vertical lines marking incisal embrasures and other landmarks are drawn on the cast.
10. Diagnostic Wax-Up:
    - A mock-up based on the proposed smile design is created on the cast and evaluated clinically. It is then tried intraorally for real-time assessment.
11. Final Adjustments:
    - Once patient approval is obtained, necessary refinements are made. Emphasis is placed on minimally invasive techniques, such as conservative tooth reduction and providing space for restorations like crowns where needed.

Section 4: Conclusion

Chapter 8:
What our Teeth says about us?

Our teeth are far more than anatomical structures—they are intimate storytellers of our lives, silently recording where we come from, how we live, and who we are. Every stain, filling, alignment, and gap reflects a tapestry of biology, behavior, culture, and evolution. Across history, civilizations have interpreted and manipulated dental features to symbolize beauty, status, power, and even spirituality. In ancient Mesoamerica, intricate tooth inlays of jade and turquoise denoted high rank; in Japanese Ohaguro, the blackening of teeth once represented loyalty and marital status.

Today, modern dentistry reads teeth like forensic clues. Enamel wear patterns can reveal a person's diet—whether they consumed hard, fibrous plants or soft, processed foods. Malocclusions may point to generational shifts in jaw size and lifestyle, while dental fluorosis or caries can reflect environmental exposure or socioeconomic conditions. Even psychological stress can leave its trace in microscopic enamel defects known as stress lines.

From the anthropologist analyzing fossilized molars to the dentist diagnosing bruxism in a teenager, teeth are a bridge between our past and present, science and society. They remind us that our smiles aren't just personal—they're profoundly human, shaped by history, and full of meaning.

Teeth as Historical Records

Teeth are remarkable structures that serve as enduring archives of human history, encapsulating intricate details about ancient diets, migrations, and health conditions. Their resilience and unique composition make them invaluable to researchers aiming to reconstruct past human experiences.

Stable Isotope Analysis and Migration Patterns

The composition of tooth enamel, particularly its stable isotope ratios, offers profound insights into the geographical origins and movements of ancient populations. Since enamel forms during early childhood and remains unchanged thereafter, it retains chemical signatures indicative of the local environment during its formation. For instance, variations in strontium and oxygen isotopes can reflect the geology and climate of a region, respectively. By analyzing these isotopes, scientists can infer whether individuals were local to an area or had migrated from elsewhere. Such analyses have been instrumental in uncovering unexpected migration patterns in ancient civilizations, challenging previous assumptions about their mobility.

Dental Calculus as a Repository of Dietary and Health Information

Dental calculus, the mineralized plaque that accumulates on teeth, encapsulates microscopic remnants of food particles, bacteria, and other substances present in the oral environment. This calcified material serves as a time capsule, preserving biomolecules that offer direct evidence of ancient diets and health conditions. Through the analysis of ancient DNA (aDNA) extracted from dental calculus, researchers have identified dietary components and oral microbiomes of past populations. For example, studies have revealed the consumption of specific plants and animals, as well as the presence of pathogens, providing a comprehensive picture of ancient lifestyles and health challenges.

Harris Lines and Indicators of Physiological Stress

Harris lines are transverse radiopaque lines visible in radiographs of long bones, indicative of temporary interruptions in bone growth, often due to physiological stress such as malnutrition or illness during childhood. While primarily observed in bones, similar stress indicators, known as enamel hypoplasias, appear in teeth. These markers provide evidence of periods when individuals experienced significant hardships, reflecting broader socio-economic and environmental conditions of their time. The presence and distribution of Harris lines and enamel hypoplasias in skeletal remains offer valuable data for understanding the health and nutritional status of ancient populations.

In essence, the study of teeth through various scientific methodologies illuminates the intricate narratives of human history, offering profound insights into the lives of our ancestors

Teeth as Identity Markers

Teeth are not only vital for mastication and aesthetics but also serve as resilient biological markers of individual identity. Their role in forensic investigations, bioarchaeology, and personal identification has made them indispensable in both historical and modern contexts. The uniqueness of dental features, their resistance to postmortem degradation, and the possibility of DNA extraction make teeth one of the most reliable tools in personal identification.

1. Uniqueness of Dental Structures

Everyone possesses a distinct dental profile, shaped by genetics, environment, dietary habits, and life experiences. Characteristics such as tooth size, shape, cusp patterns, enamel thickness, occlusal wear, and alignment contribute to a person's dental uniqueness. Even identical twins, who share the same genetic code, exhibit minor dental differences due to epigenetic and environmental factors.

Restorative dental work — including fillings, crowns, bridges, and implants — further adds to the uniqueness. These treatments are typically well documented, allowing forensic odontologists to match postmortem dental records with antemortem data, thereby confirming a person's identity with high accuracy.

2. Forensic Odontology: A Scientific Framework

Forensic odontology is a well-established discipline that uses dental records to identify unknown human remains, especially in mass disasters, criminal investigations, and cases of advanced decomposition or skeletal remains. Teeth withstand extreme environmental conditions such as fire, water submersion, or decomposition far better than soft tissues and bones, preserving identifying features for longer periods.

The American Board of Forensic Odontology and similar international bodies follow strict protocols for comparison of dental records, including analysis of dental X-rays, charts, photographic evidence, and even palatal rugae patterns. These comparisons are used in legal proceedings and have played critical roles in identifying victims in events like airplane crashes, natural disasters, and war crimes.

3. Bite Mark Analysis

Although bite mark analysis has seen increasing scrutiny in recent years due to variability in interpretation, it has historically played a significant role in criminal investigations. A suspect's dental structure— including spacing, rotations, and missing teeth — can leave unique bite impressions on victims or objects. This has been utilized to match perpetrators to specific incidents.

That said, current research encourages cautious use of bite mark evidence, recommending it as supportive rather than sole proof in legal contexts due to issues with reproducibility and subjectivity.

4. DNA Retrieval from Dental Pulp

The inner chamber of the tooth, or the pulp, is protected by hard enamel and dentin, making it an excellent reservoir for nuclear and mitochondrial DNA. This is especially valuable in cases involving unidentified remains where traditional identification methods fail. Even after years of burial or exposure to harsh environmental factors, the dental pulp can yield viable DNA for genetic profiling.

Dental DNA analysis can be used to establish kinship, solve cold cases, and confirm identities in mass fatality events. Newer techniques in forensic genomics are improving the success rates of DNA extraction from aged or damaged teeth.

5. Cultural and Anthropological Markers

In many cultures, deliberate dental modifications — such as tooth filing, ornamentation, extraction, or blackening — serve as tribal or social identifiers. These modifications often remain preserved postmortem and are significant markers in archaeological and forensic investigations.

For example, in certain African and Southeast Asian communities, front tooth removal or sharpening was (and sometimes still is) practiced as a rite of passage, identity expression, or aesthetic standard. These practices, when discovered during analysis, offer insights not only into individual identity but also their community, time period, and cultural background

Final Reflection: The Silent Storytellers of Humanity

Teeth are not merely tools of mastication or symbols of beauty; they are among the most enduring and eloquent storytellers of human existence. From our evolutionary past to forensic futures, teeth bear silent witness to where we've been, who we are, and where we are going.

Teeth as the Fossilized Timeline of Evolution

The study of dentition in hominins and other primates has revealed profound evolutionary patterns. Dental morphology—such as cusp patterns, enamel thickness, and tooth eruption sequences—helps paleoanthropologists trace the development of species, dietary adaptations, and migratory histories. Fossilized teeth provide not just structural evidence but also geochemical clues, such as isotope ratios that help determine ancient diets, environments, and even migration behaviors.

In fact, teeth are often the most intact parts of ancient skeletons due to their mineralized enamel—the hardest substance in the human body. They have survived for millions of years, giving us insights into early hominins like *Australopithecus*, *Homo erectus*, and *Neanderthals*.

Teeth as Markers of Societal Progress and Inequality

Anthropologists and sociologists have found that patterns of tooth wear, decay, and malocclusion across populations reveal much about historical lifestyles and social hierarchies. For example, industrial societies have seen a surge in dental caries due to processed sugars, while non-industrialized communities often display attritional wear from coarse diets. The presence or absence of dental care access reflects socioeconomic disparities even in modern populations, highlighting the intersection between oral health and systemic inequality.

Teeth, therefore, are not just personal records but societal mirrors, reflecting transitions in diet, health care, class, and culture.

Teeth as Connectors Between Past and Present

In the present day, teeth continue to bridge science with history. They are increasingly being used in advanced biomolecular research to extract not just human DNA, but also ancient bacterial genomes that once inhabited our mouths. This contributes to our understanding of microbiome evolution, the rise of infectious diseases, and the co-evolution of humans and pathogens.

Moreover, developments in forensic odontology and digital dentistry are using teeth to serve justice, identify disaster victims, and personalize dental care. These technological advancements enhance the role of teeth from passive indicators to active tools in shaping human outcomes.

What Our Teeth Reveal — and Conceal

Teeth reveal our diets, our diseases, our identities, and our ancestry. They encode data on environmental exposure (like lead or fluoride), periods of nutritional stress (visible in enamel hypoplasia), and even mental health conditions such as bruxism from stress. At the same time, they conceal the unspoken—trauma, survival, and adaptation—that no other organ can so discreetly preserve.

Yet, despite their durability and wealth of information, teeth can also mislead. The same dental trait can appear in unrelated individuals due to convergent evolution or cultural mimicry. Hence, while teeth are remarkable tools for understanding humanity, they must be studied in context—biological, cultural, and historical.

A Smile into the Future

As we step into the future with AI-powered diagnostics, 3D-printed prosthetics, and regenerative dental therapies, we must remember that our teeth are more than just functional assets. They are autobiographical archives—etched with evidence of our joys, pains, habits, and histories.

The smile, often considered the universal human expression, is the ultimate embodiment of what teeth represent: a blend of biology, identity, and emotion. It is in the curve of our incisor arc, the shade of our enamel, the spacing between molars, and the presence of a wisdom tooth that our story is written—not just individually, but as a species.

In the end, the study of teeth is the study of humanity itself.

If eyes are the windows to the soul, then teeth are the storytellers of our lives. Hidden behind every smile is a rich archive—etched in enamel and sealed in dentin—that speaks volumes about who we are, where we come from, and how we have evolved.

Long before written language or genetic testing, teeth were recording our biology, our behavior, and even our beliefs. They are the only parts of our bodies designed to endure long after the rest has returned to dust. Anthropologists, archaeologists, and dentists alike can look at a single molar and uncover evidence of a child's diet, a tribe's migration, a civilization's access to nutrition, or even a society's standards of beauty and health.

But teeth are not just biological artifacts—they are deeply personal. They show the stress lines from a famine endured in childhood, the wear patterns of ancient plant-based diets, or the ornamental shaping seen in certain cultures that considered tooth filing or inlays a mark of beauty and status. Through isotope analysis, scientists can now determine where a person lived as a child, even if they traveled thousands of miles before death. Through dental calculus, we can peer into the microbial world that lived inside the mouths of people who walked the Earth millennia ago.

In this sense, teeth are time travelers.

They connect the primal with the present, the scientific with the spiritual, and the anatomical with the aesthetic. A single incisor can bridge centuries of evolution—from primate ancestors to social influencers. It can symbolize power in one culture, purity in another, or even rebellion in a third. And in today's digital age, where smiles are carefully curated on screens and filters, teeth still ground us in something real—bone-deep truth, encoded in calcium and phosphate.

As we've explored in this book, the evolution of the smile is not just about how our faces have changed, but about how our values, cultures, and technologies have shaped what we consider beautiful, expressive, or meaningful. From the tooth marks in ancient bones to the digitally designed smiles of modern dentistry, our teeth have followed us through time, changing with us and adapting to reflect every chapter of human progress.

So, what do your teeth say about you?

More than just a reflection in the mirror, they are a legacy. They are your past, your present, and—thanks to advances in digital smile design and minimally invasive treatments—your future.

This book may close here, but your smile's story continues. And every time you smile, knowingly or unconsciously, you are revealing far more than emotion—you are revealing evolution.

Bibliography

1. Darwin C. *The Expression of the Emotions in Man and Animals*. London: John Murray; 1872.

2. Ungar PS. *Evolution of the Human Diet: The Known, the Unknown, and the Unknowable*. Oxford: Oxford University Press; 2006.

3. Tomasello M. *Origins of Human Communication*. Cambridge: MIT Press; 2008.

4. Strack F, Martin LL, Stepper S. Inhibiting and facilitating conditions of the human smile: A nonobtrusive test of the facial feedback hypothesis. *J Pers Soc Psychol*. 1988;54(5):768-77.

5. Matsumoto D. Cultural influences on the perception of emotion. *J Cross-Cult Psychol*. 1990;21(2):133-57.

6. Tsai JL, Chentsova-Dutton Y, Freire-Bebeau L, Przymus DE. Emotional expression and physiology in European Americans and Hmong Americans. *Emotion*. 2002;2(4):380-97.

7. Ash A. Why Japan celebrates imperfect teeth. *BBC Future* [Internet]. 2015 [cited 2025 Mar 31].

8. Proffit WR, Fields HW, Sarver DM. *Contemporary Orthodontics*. 5th ed. St. Louis: Elsevier; 2012.

9. Popenoe R. Ideal teeth: Cosmetic dentistry and consumer culture in the United States. *Med Anthropol Q*. 2004;18(4):447-67.

10. Hertenstein MJ, Hansel CA, Butts AM, Hile S. Smile intensity in photographs predicts longevity. *Psychol Sci*. 2009;20(10):1181-3.

11. Newton JT, Prabhu N, Robinson PG. The impact of dental appearance on the appraisal of personal characteristics. *Int J Prosthodont*. 2003;16(4):429-34.

12. Little AC, Jones BC, DeBruine LM. Facial attractiveness: Evolutionary based research. *Philos Trans R Soc Lond B Biol Sci*. 2011;366(1571):1638-59.

13. Dion K, Berscheid E, Walster E. What is beautiful is good. *J Pers Soc Psychol*. 1972;24(3):285-90.

14. Borkenau P, Liebler A. The halo effect: Evidence for unconscious alteration of judgments. *J Exp Soc Psychol*. 1992;28(2):137-56.

15. Belch GE, Belch MA. *Advertising and Promotion: An Integrated Marketing Communications Perspective*. 10th ed. New York: McGraw-Hill; 2017.

16. Ekman P. Facial expressions of emotion: new findings, new questions. *Psychol Sci*. 1992;3(1):34-8.

17. Rychlowska M, Jack RE, Garrod OG, Schyns PG, Martin JD, Niedenthal PM. Functional smiles: tools for love, sympathy, and war. *Psychol Sci*. 2017;28(9):1259-70.

18. Parr LA, Waller BM, Fugate J. Emotional communication in primates: implications for neurobiology. *Curr Opin Neurobiol*. 2005;15(6):716-20.

19. Keltner D, Bonanno GA. A study of laughter and dissociation: distinct correlates of laughter and smiling during bereavement. *J Pers Soc Psychol.* 1997;73(4):687-702.

20. Bugental DB, Blue J, Lewis J. Caregiver's sensitivity to young children's cues: developmental and contextual considerations. *New Dir Child Dev.* 1990;48:41-51.

21. LaFrance M, Hecht MA. Obligingsness, smiling, and gender: nonverbal behavior in compliance situations. *J Nonverbal Behav.* 1999;23:203-25.

22. Matsumoto D, Kudoh T. American-Japanese cultural differences in the recognition of universal facial expressions. *J Cross Cult Psychol.* 1993;24(4):389-410.

23. Ekman P, Friesen WV. Felt, false, and miserable smiles. *J Nonverbal Behav.* 1982;6(4):238-52.

24. Hess U, Kleck RE. Differentiating genuine from false smiles: an application of the facial action coding system. *Eur J Soc Psychol.* 1990;20(5):369-85.

25. Schneider KM, Josephs RA, Friedrich WN. Smiling in children: a developmental and situational analysis. *Dev Psychol.* 1988;24(4):465-71.

26. Matsumoto D. The role of facial response in the experience of emotion: a cross-cultural perspective. *J Nonverbal Behav.* 1987;11(3):231-43.

27. Steiner ID. Paradigms and groups. *Eur J Soc Psychol.* 1986;16(3):311-21.

28. Krause R, Steimer-Krause E. Facial expression in depressive states. *Psychopathology.* 1993;26(3-4):165-73.

29. Niedenthal PM, Brauer M, Halberstadt JB, Innes-Ker ÅH. When did her smile drop? Facial mimicry and the influences of emotional state on the detection of change in emotional expression. *Cogn Emot.* 2001;15(6):853-64.

30. Tsujimura H, Banissy MJ. Human facial expressions as a form of social communication. *Philos Trans R Soc Lond B Biol Sci.* 2013;368(1629):20120375.

31. Darwin C. *On the Origin of Species by Means of Natural Selection.* London: John Murray; 1859.
32. Hlusko LJ. Integrating the evolution of teeth and diet: insights from African primates. *Curr Opin Genet Dev.*2016;41:52-58.
33. Ungar PS. *Evolution's Bite: A Story of Teeth, Diet, and Human Origins.* Princeton University Press; 2017.
34. Nanci A. *Ten Cate's Oral Histology: Development, Structure, and Function.* 9th ed. St. Louis, MO: Elsevier; 2017.
35. Jernvall J, Thesleff I. Reiterative signaling and patterning during mammalian tooth morphogenesis. *Mech Dev.*2000;92(1):19-29.
36. Smith TM, Tafforeau P, Reid DJ, et al. Dental evidence for ontogenetic differences between modern humans and Neanderthals. *Proc Natl Acad Sci U S A.* 2010;107(49):20923-8.
37. Butler PM. Evolution of teeth and dental patterns in mammals. *Biol Rev Camb Philos Soc.* 2000;75(2):195-231.
38. Krause J, Fu Q, Good JM, et al. The complete mitochondrial DNA genome of an unknown hominin from southern Siberia. *Nature.* 2010;464(7290):894-7.
39. Berkovitz BK, Holland GR, Moxham BJ. *Oral Anatomy, Histology and Embryology.* 4th ed. Edinburgh: Mosby; 2009.
40. Balic A. Concise review: Cellular and molecular mechanisms regulating tooth initiation. *Stem Cells.* 2019;37(1):26-32.

41.
42. Soukup V, Epperlein HH, Horáček I, Cerny R. Dual epithelial origin of vertebrate oral teeth. Nature. 2008;455(7214):795-798.
43. Smith MM, Johanson Z. Origin of the vertebrate dentition: teeth transform jaws into a biting force. Science. 2003;299(5610):1235-1236.
44. Fraser GJ, Bloomquist RF, Streelman JT. Common developmental pathways link tooth shape to regeneration. Dev Biol. 2013;377(2):399-414.
45. Stock DW. The genetic basis of modularity in the development and evolution of the vertebrate dentition. Philos Trans R Soc Lond B Biol Sci. 2001;356(1414):1633-1653.
46. Donoghue PCJ, Rücklin M. The ins and outs of the evolutionary origin of teeth. Evol Dev. 2016;18(1):19-30.
47. Tucker AS, Fraser GJ. Evolution and developmental diversity of tooth regeneration. Semin Cell Dev Biol. 2014;25-26:71-80.
48. Kawasaki K, Weiss KM. Mineralized tissue and vertebrate evolution: the secretory calcium-binding phosphoprotein gene cluster. Proc Natl Acad Sci U S A. 2003;100(7):4060-4065.
49. Rücklin M, Donoghue PCJ, Johanson Z, Trinajstic K, Marone F, Stampanoni M. Developmental origins of tessellated dentition in modern sharks. Nature. 2012;491(7425):748-751.
50. Koussoulakou DS, Margaritis LH, Koussoulakos SL. A curriculum vitae of teeth: evolution, generation, regeneration. Int J Biol Sci. 2009;5(3):226-243.
51. Ungar PS. Dental evidence for the diets of fossil primates. Anat Rec (Hoboken). 2010;293(4):548-557.
52. Ungar PS. Dental evidence for the reconstruction of diet in African early Homo. *Curr Anthropol.* 2012;53(S6):S318-29.
53. Teaford MF, Ungar PS. Diet and the evolution of the human dentition: The past, present, and future of dental research. *Am J Phys Anthropol.* 2000;Suppl 31:171-91.
54. Smith TM, Toussaint M, Reid DJ, Olejniczak AJ, Hublin J-J. Rapid dental development in a Middle Paleolithic Belgian Neanderthal. *Proc Natl Acad Sci U S A.* 2007;104(51):20220-5.
55. Scott RS, Teaford MF, Ungar PS. Dental microwear texture and anthropoid diets. *Am J Phys Anthropol.*2012;147(4):551-79.
56. Grine FE. Dental evidence for dietary differences in Australopithecus and Paranthropus: A quantitative analysis of permanent molar microwear. *J Hum Evol.* 1986;15(8):783-822.
57. Aiello LC, Wheeler P. The expensive-tissue hypothesis: The brain and the digestive system in human and primate evolution. *Curr Anthropol.* 1995;36(2):199-221.
58. Ungar PS, Sponheimer M. The diets of early hominins. *Science.* 2011;334(6053):190-3.
59. Clement AF, Hillson SW. Dental microwear in modern human populations: The effects of diet, genetics and habits. *Am J Phys Anthropol.* 2013;152(3):400-10.
60. Hardy K, Buckley S, Collins MJ, Estalrrich A, Brothwell D, Copeland L, et al. Neanderthal medics? Evidence for food, cooking, and medicinal plants entrapped in dental calculus. *Naturwissenschaften.* 2012;99(8):617-26.
61. Arora M, Weuve J, Schwartz J, Wright RO. Associations of black carbon exposure with incident dental caries in primary teeth: Evidence from a birth cohort study. *Am J Public Health.* 2009;99(3):507-13.
62. Hlusko LJ, Suwa G, Kono RT. Enamel thickness and dental topography of the postcanine dentition of Australopithecus afarensis. *J Hum Evol.* 2004;46(5):571-96.
63. Perry GH, Dominy NJ, Claw KG, Lee AS, Fiegler H, Redon R, et al. Diet and the evolution of human amylase gene copy number variation. *Nat Genet.* 2007;39(10):1256-60.
64. Warinner C, Speller C, Collins MJ. A new era in palaeomicrobiology: Dental calculus and ancient disease. *Philos Trans R Soc Lond B Biol Sci.* 2015;370(1660):20130376.
65. Lucas PW, Constantino PJ, Wood B, Lawn BR. Dental enamel as a dietary indicator in mammals. *BioEssays.*2008;30(4):374-85.
66. Benazzi S, Viola B, Neubauer S, Kullmer O, Mazurier A, Ludwig K, et al. The dental roots of Homo sapiens and Neanderthals. *Sci Rep.* 2014;4:4860.

67. Eaton SB, Konner M, Shostak M. Stone agers in the fast lane: Chronic degenerative diseases in evolutionary perspective. *Am J Med.* 1988;84(4):739-49.
68. Sonnenburg ED, Sonnenburg JL. Starving our microbial self: The deleterious consequences of a diet deficient in microbiota-accessible carbohydrates. *Cell Metab.* 2014;20(5):779-86.
69. Cordain L, Eaton SB, Sebastian A, Mann N, Lindeberg S, Watkins BA, et al. Origins and evolution of the Western diet: Health implications for the 21st century. *Am J Clin Nutr.* 2005;81(2):341-54.
70. Wrangham R. Catching fire: How cooking made us human. *Basic Books*; 2009.
71. Mattson MP, Longo VD, Harvie M. Impact of intermittent fasting on health and disease processes. *Ageing Res Rev.*2017;39:46-58.
72. Kemp M. Leonardo da Vinci: The marvellous works of nature and man. Oxford University Press; 2006.
73. Livingstone MS. Is it really smiling? Vision and neuroscience in da Vinci's Mona Lisa. Science. 2000;290(5496):1145.
74. Batchen G. Forget me not: Photography and remembrance. Princeton Architectural Press; 2004.
75. Wood EM. Why didn't people smile in old photographs? BBC Future [Internet]. 2016 May 26 [cited 2025 Mar 3].
76. Gabler N. An empire of their own: How the Jews invented Hollywood. Anchor Books; 1989.
77. Karpf A. The human voice: The story of a remarkable talent. Bloomsbury Publishing; 2007.
78. Pincus DJ. The marketing of the Hollywood smile: How dentists shaped an American ideal. J Hist Dent. 2002;50(3):109-15.
79. Rychlowska M, Miyamoto Y, Matsumoto D, Hess U, Gilboa-Schechtman E, Niedenthal PM. Heterogeneity of long-history migration explains cultural differences in reports of emotional expressivity and the functions of smiles. Proc Natl Acad Sci U S A. 2015;112(19):E2429-36.
80. Matsumoto D. Cultural similarities and differences in display rules. Motiv Emot. 1990;14(3):195-214.
81. Tsai JL, Chentsova-Dutton YE, Freire-Bebeau L, Przymus DE. Emotional expression and physiology in European Americans and Hmong Americans. Emotion. 2002;2(4):380-97.
82. Danesi M. The semiotics of emoji: The rise of visual language in the age of the internet. Bloomsbury Publishing; 2017.
83. Riordan MA. Emojis as tools for emotion work: Communicating affect in text messages. J Lang Soc Psychol. 2017;36(5):549-67.
84. Luangrath AW, Peck J, Barger V. Textual paralanguage and its implications for marketing communications. J Consum Psychol. 2017;27(1):98-107.
85. Fang X, Sauter DA, van Kleef GA. Unmasking smiles: the influence of culture and intensity on interpretations of smiling expressions. J Cult Cogn Sci. 2019;3:293–308.
86.
87. Ozono H, Watabe M, Yoshikawa S, Oda R, Takahashi C, Yamagishi T. What's in a smile? Cultural differences in the effects of smiling on judgments of trustworthiness. Lett Evol Behav Sci. 2010;1(1):15-8
88. Matsumoto D, Kudoh T, Scherer KR, Wallbott HG. Cultural differences in the judgment of facial expressions: Variability or universality? J Pers Soc Psychol. 1988;54(4):768-774.

89. Hess U, Beaupré MG, Cheung N. Who to whom and why—Cultural differences and similarities in the function of smiles. In: Ambady N, Skowronski JJ, editors. The Psychology of the Social Self. Mahwah, NJ: Lawrence Erlbaum Associates; 2008. p. 187-202.

90. Rychlowska M, Miyamoto Y, Matsumoto D, Hess U, Gilboa-Schechtman E, Kamble S, et al. Heterogeneity of long-history migration explains cultural differences in reports of emotional expressivity and the functions of smiles. Proc Natl Acad Sci U S A. 2015;112(19):E2429-E2436.

91. Niedenthal PM, Rychlowska M, Wood A, Zhao F. Heterogeneity of long-history migration explains cultural differences in reports of emotional expressivity and the functions of smiles. Proc Natl Acad Sci U S A. 2015;112(19):E2429-E2436.

92. Elfenbein HA, Ambady N. On the universality and cultural specificity of emotion recognition: A meta-analysis. Psychol Bull. 2002;128(2):203-235.

93. Jack RE, Garrod OGB, Yu H, Caldara R, Schyns PG. Facial expressions of emotion are not culturally universal. Proc Natl Acad Sci U S A. 2012;109(19):7241-7244.

94. Matsumoto D. Cultural similarities and differences in display rules. Motiv Emot. 1990;14(3):195-214.

95. Tracy JL, Robins RW. The nonverbal expression of pride: Evidence for cross-cultural recognition. J Pers Soc Psychol. 2008;94(3):516-530.

96. Keltner D. Signs of appeasement: Evidence for the distinct displays of embarrassment, amusement, and shame. J Pers Soc Psychol. 1995;68(3):441-454.

97. Ekman P, Friesen WV. Constants across cultures in the face and emotion. J Pers Soc Psychol. 1971;17(2):124-129.

98. Russell JA. Is there universal recognition of emotion from facial expressions? A review of the cross-cultural studies. Psychol Bull. 1994;115(1):102-141.

99. Gendron M, Roberson D, van der Vyver JM, Barrett LF. Cultural relativity in perceiving emotion from vocalizations. Psychol Sci. 2014;25(4):911-920.

100. Yuki M, Maddux WW, Masuda T. Are the windows to the soul the same in the East and West? Cultural differences in using the eyes and mouth as cues to recognize emotions in Japan and the United States. J Exp Soc Psychol. 2007;43(2):303-311.

101. Park J, Barash GI, Levy BR. The association between culture and smiling: A meta-analytic review. J Cross Cult Psychol. 2017;48(4):498-507.

102. Hecht MA, LaFrance M. License or obligation to smile: The effect of power and sex on amount and type of smiling. Pers Soc Psychol Bull. 1998;24(12):1332-1342.

103. LaFrance M, Hecht MA, Paluck EL. The contingent smile: A meta-analysis of sex differences in smiling behavior. Psychol Bull. 2003;129(2):305-334.

104. Krys K, Vauclair CM, Capaldi CA, Lun VMC, Bond MH, Domínguez-Espinosa A, et al. Be careful where you smile: Culture shapes judgments of intelligence and honesty of smiling individuals. J Nonverbal Behav. 2016;40(2):101-116. SpringerLink

105. Matsumoto D, Willingham B. The thrill of victory and the agony of defeat: Spontaneous expressions of medal winners of the 2004 Athens Olympic Games. J Pers Soc Psychol. 2009;96(3):568-576.

106. Hess U, Thibault P. Darwin and emotion expression. Am Psychol. 2009;64(2):120-128.

107. Crivelli C, Russell JA. Facial expressions in a remote indigenous society: Lack of recognition of Western facial expressions of emotion. Emotion. 2014;14(2):373-387.

108. Gendron M, Roberson D, van der Vyver JM, Barrett LF. Perceptions of emotion from facial expressions are not culturally universal: Evidence from a remote culture. Emotion. 2014;14(2):251-262.

109. Haidt J, Keltner D. Culture and facial expression: Open-ended methods find more expressions and a gradient of recognition. Cogn Emot. 1999;13(3):225-266.

110. Matsumoto D, Yoo SH, Fontaine J. Mapping expressive differences around the world: The relationship between emotional display rules and individualism versus collectivism. J Cross Cult Psychol. 2008;39(1):55-74.

111. Tsai JL, Chentsova-Dutton Y, Freire-Bebeau L, Przymus DE. Emotional expression and physiology in European American and Hmong American women. Emotion. 2002;2(4):380-397.

112. Sauter DA, Eisner F, Ekman P, Scott SK. Cross-cultural recognition of basic emotions through nonverbal emotional vocalizations. Proc Natl Acad Sci U S A. 2010

113. Niedenthal, P. M. (2007). Embodied emotion. *Current Directions in Psychological Science*, 16(4), 193-197.

114. Kershaw, S., Newton, J. T., & Williams, D. M. (2008). The influence of tooth color on perceptions of personal characteristics. *Am J Orthod Dentofacial Orthop*, 133(3), 389-394.
115. Soussignan, R. (2002). Duchenne smile, emotional experience, and autonomic reactivity: A test of the facial feedback hypothesis. *Emotion*, 2(1), 52-74.
116. Klages, U., Claus, N., Wehrbein, H., & Zentner, A. (2004). Psychosocial impact of dental aesthetics. *Eur J Orthod*, 26(1), 65-72.
117. Pithon, M. M., et al. (2014). Do dental esthetics have any influence on finding a job? *Am J Orthod Dentofacial Orthop*, 146(4), 423-429.
118. Shulman, J. D., & Brehm, W. T. (2008). The effects of dental condition on job interview outcomes. *Am J Public Health*, 98(12), 2176-2180.
119. Newton, J. T., Prabhu, N., & Robinson, P. G. (2003). Impact of dental appearance on appraisal of personal characteristics. *Int J Prosthodont*, 16(4), 429-434.
120. Samorodnitzky-Naveh, G. R., et al. (2010). Self-esteem and dental anomalies. *Eur J Oral Sci*, 118(6), 588-592.
121. Dumitrescu, A. L., Zetu, L., & Teslaru, S. (2009). Psychological aspects of anterior tooth loss. *Oral Health Prev Dent*, 7(1), 45-51.
122. Agou, S., et al. (2011). Self-esteem and malocclusion in children. *Am J Orthod Dentofacial Orthop*, 140(3), 387-392.
123. Phillips, C., Beal, K., & White, R. P. (1997). Self-concept and orthodontic treatment. *Am J Orthod Dentofacial Orthop*, 112(6), 630-639.
124. Afroz, S., Rathi, S. K., Rajput, G., & Rahman, S. A. (2013). Dental aesthetics and self-perception. *J Int Soc Prev Community Dent*, 3(1), 62-65.
125. Gerritsen, A. E., et al. (2010). Oral health and quality of life. *Gerodontology*, 27(1), 3-8.

126. Coachman, C., et al. (2017). Digital Smile Design: A new era in dentistry. *J Esthet Restor Dent*, 29(3), 192-202.

127. Pithon, M. M., et al. (2014). Influence of dental esthetics on job prospects. *Am J Orthod Dentofacial Orthop*, 146(4), 423-429.

128. Sadangi B, Nayak L, Panda PC. Traditional phytotherapy for ear, nose and throat (ENT) diseases in Kalahandi district of Odisha, India. *Indian Journal of Traditional Knowledge*. 2013;12(4):682-8.

129. Jadhav D. Traditional ethnomedicinal knowledge for the treatment of fever in Maharashtra, India. *International Journal of Green Pharmacy*. 2013;7(4):288–92.

130. Kadel C, Jain AK. Ethnomedicinal studies of the flora in Madhya Pradesh and Chhattisgarh, India. *Ethnobotany*. 2008;20:49–53.

131. Kumar N, Vivek N, Kumar V, Kumar A. Medicinal plants used in dentistry: A review. *Journal of Indian Academy of Oral Medicine and Radiology*. 2013;25(1):13–8.

132. Gurib-Fakim A. Medicinal plants: Traditions of yesterday and drugs of tomorrow. *Mol Aspects Med*. 2006;27(1):1–93. doi:10.1016/j.mam.2005.07.008

133. Fabricant DS, Farnsworth NR. The value of plants used in traditional medicine for drug discovery. *Environ Health Perspect*. 2001;109(Suppl 1):69–75. doi:10.1289/ehp.01109s169

134. Satyavati GV, Gupta AK, Tandon N. *Medicinal Plants of India*. Vol. 2. New Delhi: Indian Council of Medical Research; 1987.

135. Kaur R, Kapoor R, Kaur H. Traditional herbal remedies used for oral health care in India: A review. *Journal of Medicinal Plants Studies*. 2015;3(6):29–32.

136. Almas K. The antimicrobial effects of seven different types of Asian chewing sticks. *Odontostomatol Trop*. 2001;24(96):17–20.

137. Sofrata A, Claesson R, Lingström P, Gustafsson A. Strong antibacterial effect of miswak against oral microorganisms associated with periodontitis and caries. *J Periodontol*. 2008;79(8):1474–9. doi:10.1902/jop.2008.080109

138. Grover HS, Luthra S, Maroo S, Gupta A, Saksena S. Herbal medicine in dentistry. *J Indian Acad Oral Med Radiol*. 2011;23(3):271–6.

139. Bhushan B, Sardana D, Bansal K. Neem in dentistry: A mini review. *J Adv Med Dent Scie Res*. 2014;2(3):89–92.

140. Ananthanarayan R, Paniker CKJ. *Textbook of Microbiology*. 9th ed. Hyderabad: Universities Press; 2013. (for traditional antibacterial mechanisms)

141. Palombo EA. Traditional medicinal plant extracts and natural products with activity against oral bacteria: Potential application in the prevention and treatment of oral diseases. *Evid Based Complement Alternat Med*. 2011;2011:680354. doi:10.1093/ecam/neq035

142. Pandey R, Rathod V, Nema RK. Chewing sticks in dentistry: A review. *J Oral Health Comm Dent*. 2008;2(2):29–32.

143. Rahmani AH, Aldebasi YH. Potential role of medicinal plants in oral health care. *Asian J Pharm Clin Res*. 2013;6(Suppl 1):5–9.

144. Sushruta Samhita. *English translation of Sushruta Samhita by Kunjalal Bhishagratna*. Vol. 2. Varanasi: Chowkhamba Sanskrit Series Office; 2008.

145. Tripathi KD. *Essentials of Medical Pharmacology*. 7th ed. New Delhi: Jaypee Brothers Medical Publishers; 2013. (for pharmacology of traditional extracts)

146. Arweiler NB, Netuschil L. The oral microbiota. *Adv Exp Med Biol*. 2016;902:45–60. doi:10.1007/5584_2015_5002

147. Pundir RK, Jain P, Sharma C. Antimicrobial activity of ethanolic extracts of Syzygium cumini and Ocimum sanctum against oral pathogens. *J Pharm Bioallied Sci*. 2010;2(4):360–3. doi:10.4103/0975-7406.72134

148. Balappanavar AY, Sardana V, Singh M. Herbal oral care products: A review. *Indian J Dent Res*. 2013;24(5):697–700. doi:10.4103/0970-9290.123374

149. Ghalioungui P. *The Ebers Papyrus: A New English Translation, Commentaries and Glossaries*. Cairo: Academy of Scientific Research and Technology; 1987.

150. Breasted JH. *The Edwin Smith Surgical Papyrus*. Chicago: University of Chicago Press; 1930.

151. Filer J. Disease. In: Shaw I, editor. *The Oxford History of Ancient Egypt*. Oxford: Oxford University Press; 2000. p. 338–9.

152. Dawson WR, Gray PHK. *Catalogue of the Egyptian Antiquities in the British Museum. Vol II: Mummies and Human Remains*. London: British Museum; 1968.

153. Nunn JF. *Ancient Egyptian Medicine*. London: British Museum Press; 1996.

154. Hillson S. *Dental Anthropology*. Cambridge: Cambridge University Press; 1996.

155. Leek FF. The dental remains. In: Gray PHK, editor. *The Anatomy of the Egyptians*. London: Duckworth; 1980.

156. Blustein R, El-Etr HA, Szymanski C. The history of dentistry in ancient Egypt. *Bull Hist Dent*. 1991;39(2):9–14.

157. Nickol ME, Zivie A. A possible dental prosthesis from Saqqara: Re-evaluation of a "bridge" from ancient Egypt. *Br Dent J*. 2009;206(11):E20. doi:10.1038/sj.bdj.2009.355.

158. Hooton EA. Oral surgery in Egypt during the Old Empire. *Am Anthropol*. 1917;19(4):482–6.

159. Bass WM. *Human Osteology: A Laboratory and Field Manual*. 4th ed. Columbia: Missouri Archaeological Society; 1995.

160. Abdel-Halim RE. Contributions of medieval Islamic medicine to modern dentistry. *Saudi Dent J*. 2014;26(2):55–60. doi:10.1016/j.sdentj.2013.12.002.

161. Pincus, C. R. (1938). *Building Mouth Personality*. The Journal of the California Dental Association.

162. Goldstein, R. E. (2009). *Change Your Smile: Discover How a New Smile Can Transform Your Life*. Quintessence Publishing.

163. Morley, J. (2001). The role of cosmetic dentistry in restoring a youthful appearance. *The Journal of the American Dental Association*, 132(1), 51–58.

164. Christensen, G. J. (2007). The advantages of minimally invasive dentistry. *The Journal of the American Dental Association*, 138(5), 621–625.

165. American Academy of Cosmetic Dentistry (AACD). (2020). *History of Cosmetic Dentistry.*

166. Goldstein, R. E. (2009). *Change Your Smile*. Quintessence Publishing.

167. Spear FM, Kokich VG. A multidisciplinary approach to esthetic dentistry in: successful esthetic and cosmetic dentistry for the modern dental practice. Dent Clin North Am. 2007;51:299–318. doi: 10.1016/j.cden.2006.12.007. [DOI] [PubMed] [Google Scholar]

168. Bhuvaneswaran M. Principles of smile design. J Conserv Dent. 2010;13:225–32. doi: 10.4103/0972-0707.73387. [DOI] [PMC free article] [PubMed] [Google Scholar]
169. Dawson PE. Determining the determinants of occlusion. Int J Periodontics Restorative Dent. 1983;3:8–21. [PubMed] [Google Scholar]
170. Godara M, Khetarpal A, Rana M, Joon A, Vijayran K, Singhal N. Smile esthetic: A review. IOSR J Dent Med Sci (IOSR-JDMS) 2021;20:17–22. [Google Scholar]
171. Aschheim KW. Esthetic dentistry: a clinical approach to techniques and materials. Elsevier Health Sciences. 2014 [Google Scholar]
172. Rubin LR, Mishriki Y, Lee G. Anatomy of the nasolabial fold: The keystone of the smiling mechanism. Plast Reconstr Surg. 1989;83:1–10. doi: 10.1097/00006534-198901000-00001. [DOI] [PubMed] [Google Scholar]
173. Ackerman JL, Ackerman MB, Brensinger CM, Landis JR. A morphometric analysis of the posed smile. Clin Orth Res. 1998;1:2–11. doi: 10.1111/ocr.1998.1.1.2. [DOI] [PubMed] [Google Scholar]
174. Ackerman MB, Ackerman JL. Smile analysis and design in the digital era. J Clin Orthod. 2002;36:221–36. [PubMed] [Google Scholar]
175. Goldstein RE. Smile analysis and design in the digital era. J Clin Orthod. 2002;36:221–36.[PubMed] [Google Scholar]
176. Lavere AM. Denture tooth selection: An analysis of the natural maxillary central incisor compared to the length and width of the face. Part I. J Prosthet Dent. 1992;67:661–3. doi: 10.1016/0022-3913(92)90166-8. [DOI] [PubMed] [Google Scholar]
177. Sabri R. The eight components of a balanced smile. J Clin Orthod. 2005;39:155–67. quiz 154.[PubMed] [Google Scholar]
178. Ricketts RM. The biological significance of the divine proportion and Fibonacci Series. Am J Orthod. 1982;81:351–70. doi: 10.1016/0002-9416(82)90073-2. [DOI] [PubMed] [Google Scholar]
179. Levin EI. Dental aesthetics and Golden proportion. J Prosthet Dent. 1978;40:244–52. doi: 10.1016/0022-3913(78)90028-8. [DOI] [PubMed] [Google Scholar]
180. Kokich VG, Spear FM, Kokich VO. Maximizing anterior aesthetics: A multidisciplinary approach to esthetic dentistry. Dental Clinics of North America. 2007;51:487–505. doi: 10.1016/j.cden.2006.12.007. [DOI] [PubMed] [Google Scholar]
181. Evolution of Smile Design. [Last accessed on 2021 Aug 05]. Available from: https://media.digitalsmiledesign.com/christian-coachman-thoughts/smile-design-evolution .
182. Graber LW, Vanarsdall RL, Vig KW, Huang GJ. Orthodonticse- book: current principles and techniques. Elsevier Health Sciences. 2016 [Google Scholar]
183. Sarver DM, Ackerman MB. Dynamic smile visualization and quantification: part 1. Evolution of the concept and dynamic records for smile capture. American journal of orthodontics and dentofacial orthopedics. 2003;124:4–12. doi: 10.1016/s0889-5406(03)00306-8. [DOI] [PubMed] [Google Scholar]

184. Singla S, Lehl G. Smile analysis in orthodontics. Indian J Oral Sci. 2014;5:49–54. [Google Scholar]
185. Coachman C, Yoshinaga L, Calamita M, Sesma N. Digital smile design concepts. The Technologist. 2014 [Google Scholar]
186. Coachman C, Calamita M. Digital smile design: A tool for treatment planning and communication in aesthetic dentistry. Quintessence Dent Technol. 2012;35:103–11. [Google Scholar]
187. McLaren EA, Garber DA, Figueira J. The Photoshop Smile Design technique (part 1): Digital dental photography. Compend Contin Educ Dent. 2013;34:772, 774, 776 passim. [PubMed] [Google Scholar]
188. Gupta C, Mittal A. Role of digital technology in prosthodontics: A step toward improving dental care. Indian J Oral Health Res. 2018;4:35–41. [Google Scholar]
189. Jafri Z, Ahmad N, Sawai M, Sultan N, Bhardwaj A. Digital Smile Design-An innovative tool in aesthetic dentistry. J Oral Biol Craniofac Res. 2020;10:194–8. doi: 10.1016/j.jobcr.2020.04.010.[DOI] [PMC free article] [PubMed] [Google Scholar]
190. Coachman C, Calamita M, Ricci A. Ronald E, editor. Digital Smile Design: A Digital tool for esthetic evaluation, team communication, and patient management. Goldstein's Esthetics in Dentistry. 2018:84–111. [Google Scholar]
191. Aragón ML, Pontes L, Bichara L, Flores-Mir C, Normando D. Validity and reliability of intraoral scanners compared to conventional gypsum models measurements: A systematic review. Eur J Orthod. 2016;38:429–34. doi: 10.1093/ejo/cjw033. [DOI] [PubMed] [Google Scholar]
192. Ilić DV, Stojanović LS. Application of radiovisiography (digital radiology) in dental clinical practice. Vojnosanit Pregl. 2012;69:81–4. [PubMed] [Google Scholar]
193. Larsen CS. Bioarchaeology: Interpreting Behavior from the Human Skeleton. 2nd ed. Cambridge University Press; 2015.

194. Bentley RA. Strontium isotopes from the earth to the archaeological skeleton: a review. *Journal of Archaeological Method and Theory*. 2006;13(3):135-187.

195. Cucina A, Tiesler V. Dental decoration and pathology in Classic Maya elite: A bioarchaeological study. *Latin American Antiquity*. 2003;14(3):343–358.

196. Warinner C, Hendy J, Speller C, et al. Direct evidence of milk consumption from ancient human dental calculus. *Scientific Reports*. 2014;4:7104.

197. Pretty IA, Sweet D. A look at forensic dentistry – Part 1: The role of teeth in the determination of human identity. *British Dental Journal*. 2001;190(7):359-366.

198. Scott GR, Irish JD. Human Tooth Crown and Root Morphology: The Arizona State University Dental Anthropology System. Cambridge University Press; 2017.

199. Pretty IA, Sweet D. A look at forensic dentistry – Part 1: The role of teeth in the determination of human identity. *Br Dent J.* 2001;190(7):359-66.

200. Sweet D, Hildebrand D. Recovery of DNA from human teeth by cryogenic grinding. *J Forensic Sci.* 1998;43(6):1199-202.

201. Bowers CM, Bell GL. Digital analysis of bite mark evidence using Adobe Photoshop. *Am J Forensic Med Pathol.*1999;20(3):233–9.

202. American Board of Forensic Odontology. Diplomate reference manual. 2019.

203. Pretty IA, Sweet D. The scientific basis for human bite mark analyses – a critical review. *Sci Justice.* 2001;41(2):85-92.

204. Saks MJ, Koehler JJ. The coming paradigm shift in forensic identification science. *Science.* 2005;309(5736):892–5.

205. Malaver AL, Yunis JJ. Different dental tissues as source of DNA for human identification in forensic cases. *Croat Med J.* 2003;44(3):306–9.

206. Higgins D, Austin JJ. Teeth as a source of DNA for forensic identification of human remains: A review. *Sci Justice.*2013;53(4):433–41.

207. Alt KW, Pichler S. Cultural modification of the teeth. In: Alt KW, Rosing FW, Teschler-Nicola M, editors. *Dental Anthropology: Fundamentals, Limits, and Prospects.* Vienna: Springer; 1998. p. 479–500.

208. Teschler-Nicola M. Dental modification and mutilation: anthropology and forensic implications. *Anthropol Anz.*1995;53(3):231–50.

209. Bailey SE, Wood BA. Hominin dental evolution: Current trends and new directions. *Evol Anthropol.* 2007;16(3):93–103.

210. Ungar PS, Sponheimer M. The diets of early hominins. *Science.* 2011;334(6053):190–3.

211. Smith TM, Tafforeau P. New visions of dental development in human evolution. *Evolutionary Anthropology: Issues, News, and Reviews.* 2008;17(5):213–26.

212. Larsen CS. Bioarchaeology: Interpreting Behavior from the Human Skeleton. 2nd ed. Cambridge: Cambridge University Press; 2015.

213. Watt RG, Sheiham A. Inequalities in oral health: A review of the evidence and recommendations for action. *Br Dent J.*1999;187(1):6–12.

214. Adler CJ, Dobney K, Weyrich LS, et al. Sequencing ancient calcified dental plaque shows changes in oral microbiota with dietary shifts of the Neolithic and Industrial revolutions. *Nat Genet.* 2013;45(4):450–5.

215. Acharya AB, Taylor JA. Are a minimum number of skeletal traits necessary to establish positive forensic identification? *J Forensic Sci.* 2003;48(3):543–9.

216. Goodman AH, Rose JC. Assessment of systemic physiological perturbations from dental enamel hypoplasias and associated histological structures. *Yearbook of Physical Anthropology.* 1990;33:59–110